HOW PROFESSIONALS

*E*XPLORE
*T*RANSFORM
*F*LOURISH

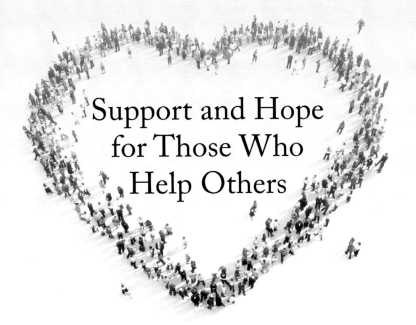

Support and Hope
for Those Who
Help Others

POWERED BY

BOOKS

GILLIAN STEVENS

Copyright © MMXVII Gillian Stevens

ALL RIGHTS RESERVED. No part of this book may be reproduced or transmitted in any form whatsoever, electronic, or mechanical, including photocopying, recording, or by any informational storage or retrieval system without the expressed written, dated and signed permission from the author.

Author: Gillian Stevens
Title: Explore, Transform, Flourish
ISBN: 978-1-77204-837-7
Category: SELF-HELP/Personal Growth/Happiness

Publisher: Black Card Books
Division of Gerry Robert Enterprises Inc.
Suite 214, 5-18 Ringwood Drive
Stouffville, Ontario, Canada, L4A 0N2
International Calling: +1 877 280 8536
www.blackcardbooks.com

....

LIMITS OF LIABILITY/DISCLAIMER OF WARRANTY: The author and publisher of this book have used their best efforts in preparing this material. The author and publisher disclaim any warranties (expressed or implied), or merchantability for any particular purpose. The author and publisher shall in no event be held liable for any loss or other damages, including, but not limited to special, incidental, consequential, or other damages. The information presented in this publication is compiled from sources believed to be accurate at the time of printing, however, the publisher assumes no responsibility for errors or omissions. The information in this publication is not intended to replace or substitute professional advice. The author and publisher specifically disclaim any liability, loss, or risk that is incurred as a consequence, directly or indirectly, of the use and application of any of the contents of this information.

Black Card Books bears no responsibility for the accuracy of information on any websites cited and/or used by the author in this book. The inclusion of website addresses in this book does not constitute an endorsement by, or associate Black Card Books with such sites or the content, products, advertising or other materials presented.

Opinions expressed by the author do not necessarily represent the views and opinions of Black Card Books. The publisher assumes no liability for any content or opinion expressed by, or through the author.

Printed in Canada

DEDICATION

To Kayla, Miranda and Graeme, who are my greatest gifts and teachers. It has been my pleasure and honour to be your mother and watch with pride as you courageously pursue your dreams and obtain success wherever you place your focus.

To us: As human beings, may we have the courage to follow our hearts, pursue our dreams and lead a flourishing life.

> "The plain fact is that the planet does not need more successful people. But it does desperately need more peacemakers, healers, restorers, storytellers, and lovers of every kind."
>
> —DAVID ORR

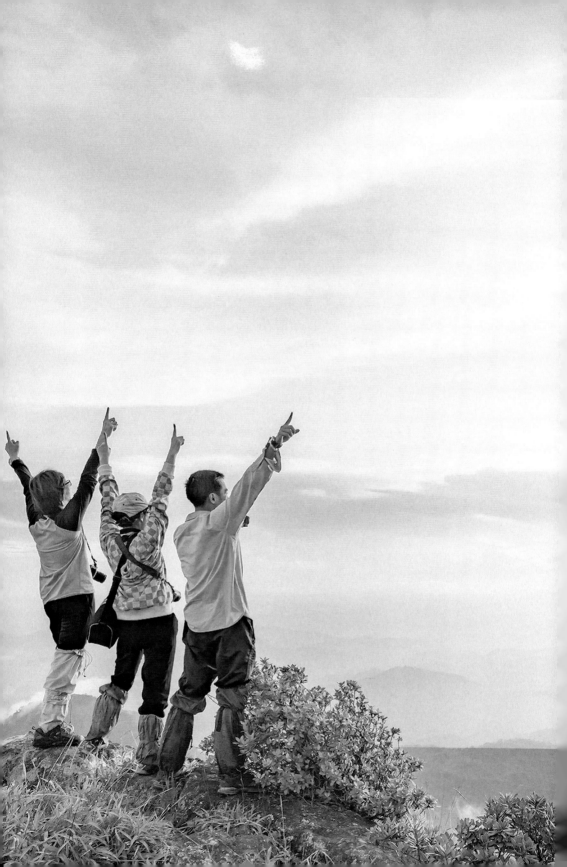

TABLE *of* CONTENTS

Testimonials

Introduction: Keeping It Together? 01

Part One: Explore

Chapter One: You Get What You Think About 13

Chapter Two: Love Is an Action Word 31

Chapter Three: Stuck in a Rut, or Are You? 49

Part Two: Transform

Chapter Four: Dancing as Fast as I Can 63

Chapter Five: Starting with the (Woman) Man in the Mirror 77

Chapter Six: Don't Die with Your Music Still Inside You 85

Part Three: Flourish

Chapter Seven: All Is Well 95

Chapter Eight: The Choice Is Yours 107

End Notes: Nothing Moves Until You Do 114

Acknowledgements 119

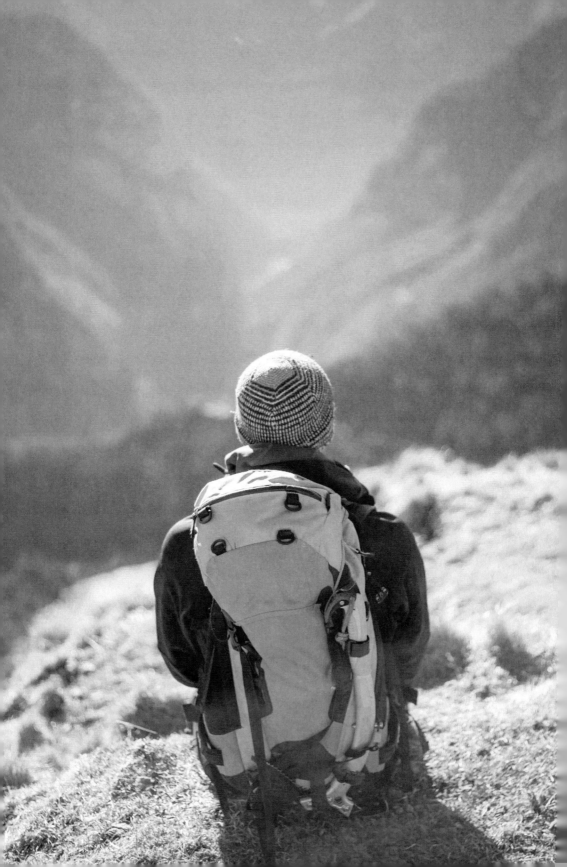

TESTIMONIALS

"Working with Gillian Stevens for more than 10 years, I observed and admired a Guidance Counsellor and Student Success Teacher who brought positive energy and honesty every day. Gillian's direct approach and straightforward inquiry paved the way for students, families and staff to deal with school difficulties, disappointment and grief. Gillian's specialty is helping people take steps towards a fresh start. Countless students have shared how much Ms. Stevens believed in them and how she 'saved' them when they needed it most. Gillian's expertise in dealing with loss and grief opened the door for students and staff to have heartfelt conversations for both simple and complex situations.

Gillian's gift is her ability to cut through the fog and get to the essence of the problem. Gillian's words of encouragement include simple steps to put personal healing first. Gillian's students and friends learn to feel empowered with purposeful self-care as the starting point for problem solving.

Gillian has been my friend and accountability partner over the last few years as I have had to deal with complicated grief. Gillian's compassion, empathy and words of guidance focused on self-care and intentional healing have been the light that helps make the darkness and sadness not as frightening."

—Linda Adams, Former Head of Student Services, CWDHS

TESTIMONIALS

"Gillian is a well-polished speaker with a clear message and excellent knowledge regarding the impact of working with people and professionals in their various roles. Her presentation leaves the audience challenged and contemplating changes they would benefit from in their lives."

—Wendy Lantz, MSW, RSW, Organizer for Social Work Week, Kitchener

---

"For as long as I have known Gillian (more than 15 years), she has been driven with a singular passion to help.

Life has provided many opportunities and that path has not always been easy, such as the challenges that come with being the sole provider to three amazing children. However, Gillian has met each of these challenges with grace, never losing hope, having faith that each experience would provide her with the wisdom to carry forward.

This book is a culmination of years of reflection, wisdom, faith and passion. Gillian's words are given in love, wrapped in faith and hope and when followed will provide helpers with a guide to care for themselves as they help others."

—Merrilynn Downey, Kilbride and Associates

"Gillian's recent presentation, to my class of teacher candidates, on student success and compassion fatigue was engaging, highly informative, timely and very well received by the teacher candidates. Gillian's ability to communicate respect for her audience and admiration for their choice of a helping profession instantly built a positive rapport and created a learning atmosphere.

Gillian's passion for student success was infectious. Her deep professional expertise helped the candidates see the need to reach out and connect with every student regardless of background, behaviour or circumstance, so the students could have a sense of belonging and have a chance for success. Teacher candidates were reminded of their power to either uplift or harm students, simply by their choice of words or actions.

Gillian's fresh perspective on the challenges of teaching and the realities of having students, who have experienced trauma in every class, resonated with the teacher candidates. She helped them to reflect on previous experiences, consider their actions, recognize signs of trauma and understand the impact of trauma on learning and students' futures.

Gillian's highly relevant perspective on compassion fatigue addressed the teacher candidates facing their own struggles with stress and feelings of being overwhelmed. Students felt heard and re-affirmed and Gillian helped them understand the importance for self-care before they could help others.

Overall, the teacher candidates felt informed and more prepared for their placements after hearing Gillian's presentation. It is without any hesitation I recommend Gillian's presentation for teacher candidates, practicing teachers or any one working in a helping profession."

—Deidre Wilson, Sessional Instructor, Brock University

Additional testimonials from students:

"She is clearly very knowledgeable about the topic and shows her passion for making sure all students succeed."

"Gave me a lot of insight for grief and how important it is to help ourselves, in order to fully be better and able to support our students."

"Grief and trauma is not talked about enough. It is important to be reminded to take care of ourselves first."

"Very insightful woman, very fluent and confident in her speaking. The information really stuck with me especially about how students can be dealing with trauma and the huge effect it can have on the student's future."

"This presentation made me consider experiences I have had in a new way and really opened my eyes to mistakes or misunderstandings I have made in the past."

"Highly sensitive people are too often perceived as weaklings or damaged goods. To feel intensely is not a symptom of weakness; it is the trademark of the truly alive and compassionate. It is not the empath who is broken; it is society that has become dysfunctional and emotionally disabled. There is no shame in expressing your authentic feelings. Those who are at times described as being a 'hot mess' or having 'too many issues' are the very fabric of what keeps the dream alive for a more caring, humane world. Never be ashamed to let your tears shine a light in this world."

—ANTHON ST. MAARTEN

INTRODUCTION:
Keeping It Together?

In the words of Dr. Phil, "How's this working for you?" It wasn't working for me; I was keeping it together until I couldn't. Does keeping it together mean we soldier on, handling the many demands on our time even when we are not happy and experiencing vague physical symptoms that, if ignored, could potentially become serious? We know it's important to take care of ourselves, and yet it has become accepted practice to sacrifice our health and what we want and need. Life is busier than it's ever been and there seems to be an unspoken reward or validation the busier you are. Many of us, me included, went into our careers to help others, and because we wanted to make a difference in someone's life. We have become so distracted with the issues of the world that we have forgotten to take care of ourselves.

In his book *Future Shock*, Alvin Toffler said, "Change is happening so quickly and information becoming so voluminous that people wouldn't be able to handle it emotionally and society will suffer if steps aren't taken to better prepare for change." When we are exposed to rapid change and fear, we are not keeping it together; we experience feelings of helplessness and inadequacy. We have feelings of insecurity and worry about the state of the world, our economic future and the threat of job loss due to cutbacks and downsizing and anxiety is prevalent in our society.

> To cope and succeed, we need to be able to adapt, quickly. We constantly need to relearn what is now relevant in our jobs, our careers and in our lives and let go of or "unlearn" old ways.

INTRODUCTION: KEEPING IT TOGETHER?

There is a generalized feeling of anxiety that exists based on a feeling that bad things may happen, and this is often reinforced by trauma we witness or hear about in our jobs, which further heightens our anxiety. The anxiety and fear we feel is the stress response, fight or flight, and our body is flooded with cortisol and adrenaline. Another response to stress is to freeze, which is identified with numbing, apathy, despair and depression. These two stress responses can lead to burnout, depression and drug addiction due to feelings of helplessness. If we can't find a way to manage unpredictable and uncontrollable change, we experience loss of control and distress, which can also result in anxiety, apathy and depression.

To cope and succeed, we need to be able to adapt, quickly. We constantly need to relearn what is now relevant in our jobs, our careers and in our lives and let go of or "unlearn" old ways. Unlearning is about being open to and exploring new ideas by letting go of our conditioning. Learning agility is the key to success in a constantly changing environment both personally and professionally.

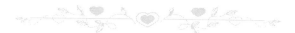

"The illiterate of the 21st century will not be those who cannot read and write, but those who cannot learn, unlearn, and relearn."

—ALVIN TOFFLER

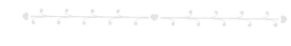

We seem to be at a crisis point, given the rising incidences of burnout, compassion fatigue, post-traumatic stress disorder, suicides, opiate addiction and so on. Diagnoses of breast cancer are also on the rise, which I find interesting as the breast is symbolic of nourishing and taking care of others, and it appears we are doing so to our detriment.

We soldier on day after day, exposed to our clients' pain and suffering and often feeling powerless to effect change in them and the systems in which we work. The demands of our job are growing; we are asked to do more with less and see more clients daily who are presenting with more complex issues.

Dr. Joan Borysenko, author of *Fried: Why You Burn Out and How to Revive*, describes burnout as a spiritual crisis where "our sense of meaning and purpose has disappeared from view and we don't know which way to turn". She further states that burnout is "the malady of the times, which manifests in depression-like symptoms and the physical symptoms of extreme stress, which includes digestive shutdown, inflammation, adrenal fatigue and a compromised immune system". Dr. Jane Simington of Taking Flight International, who provides training in trauma recovery, suicide intervention and grief support, similarly suggests burnout is more than overwork. She says it is "an erosion of the soul and the soul's need to be living the life you were meant to live, accompanied by the feeling that regardless of what you do you cannot make a difference in the workplace". Dr. Frank Lipman, author of *Revive: Stop Feeling Spent and Start Living Again*, suggests that burnout is a common concern. The fast pace of our lives creates the problem, and with our cultural and environmental stressors, we just never turn off.

Whether we are talking about burnout, compassion fatigue or any of the stress-related conditions of epidemic proportions, they are the effects of an imbalance and our body's (mind, heart and spirit) inability to cope. It's obvious that what we are doing isn't working, and we are being invited to address the cause of our body's dis-ease related to these rapidly changing times. In support of both Borysenko and Simington, I believe we need to be alert to what our body and soul need and ask the questions: Are we living the life we are meant to be living? What are my body symptoms and intuition trying to tell me?

INTRODUCTION: KEEPING IT TOGETHER?

"If something is not working, doing more of it will not work any better."

—ANONYMOUS

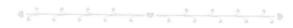

Who Are "We"?

According to Wiktionary, a helping profession is "a profession that nurtures the growth of or addresses the problems of a person's physical, psychological, intellectual, emotional and spiritual well-being including medicine, nursing, social work, psychotherapy, counselling, education, life coaching and ministry". Many of us are bearing the responsibilities of raising children and supporting our parents in addition to our jobs. We are all helpers and professionals doing the best we can in the work we do: Volunteering, caregiving, parenting and supporting our parents.

Who Am I?

I am a caregiver, coach, teacher, parent and counsellor. I took a semester leave from teaching early in my career due to the stress of an acrimonious separation and the ongoing struggle to secure a full-time teaching position while raising three young children with limited to no child support. I realized that my health had to be of the utmost importance, as I was solely responsible for our children and their well-being. To help them, I had to help myself first.

I returned to teaching the following semester and eventually moved into a role in the guidance department, where I worked with students who were at risk of not graduating. Some of the barriers to their success were mental health issues, family dynamics, poverty, substance abuse, attendance concerns and lack of engagement within the system. I also recognized that many of them had unresolved grief related to loss, which caused them a great deal of emotional pain.

As the years crept on, I became disheartened and frustrated within a system that seemed unwilling to proactively support all elementary students in developing interpersonal skills and develop the grit necessary for success in school and life. Instead, we chose to be reactive in our approach, supporting fewer students with more significant issues at the secondary level—work that was challenging due to limited resources. I wanted desperately to make a difference, but there were many obstacles in my way and I felt stuck. Finally, I came to the decision to retire early and focus on what I could do from a more positive perspective.

The decision to retire was difficult as I enjoyed working with the students, my colleagues and until recent years had experienced a positive and supportive working relationship with my school administration. In the last few years, however, I felt my administration was not supportive nor appreciative of both my experience and skill set and that affected my attitude and health. I felt I had no choice but to leave my job. Over the years, I had the opportunity to interact with many teachers, parents, counsellors and administrators with the sole task of helping students, and through conversations with those individuals, I realized I wasn't the only one affected by the challenges of working in a helping profession. Once I announced my retirement, writing this book seemed the logical next step. I could make a difference by writing a book that supported those who give of their time and energy to help others while often sacrificing their own well-being and needs and desires.

In retrospect, it all worked out perfectly. Instead of feeling I had no choice but to leave, I shifted my perception to believing I made the choice to leave and pursue my dream of being a writer. I began to

INTRODUCTION: KEEPING IT TOGETHER?

feel grateful for my previous circumstances and recognized it was in my best interest to leave the teaching profession and write this book. The obstacle I thought was in the way actually became the way as expressed in Marcus Aurelius' quote, "The impediment to action advances the action. What stands in the way becomes the way." Brian Johnson of Optimize +1 expanded further on this quote and offers these questions to ponder as a way of maintaining a positive focus and motivation when encountering challenges.

> As the obstacles surface on your path of change, which inevitably they will, remember they are the way. Rub your hands together and go for it with excitement and enthusiasm.

What if we just let the obstacle BE the way?

What if we trained ourselves to immediately accept and love what it is as we rub our hands together at the opportunity to create a better plan using this new variable as a catalyst and go from there?

As I did final edits on this section of my book, I realized that the many challenges I encountered while writing this book were actually the obstacles that became the way to not only improving the content of the book through personal growth but also to creating a flourishing life. As the obstacles surface on your path of change, which inevitably they will, remember they are the way. Rub your hands together and go for it with excitement and enthusiasm.

"If you believe it will work out, you'll see opportunities. If you believe it won't, you will see obstacles."

—WAYNE DYER

What Did I Discover?

I initially began gathering the content for the book by interviewing people who worked in education and social work. Next, I interviewed first responders, and that led me to extending my reach and interviewing individuals in the financial and insurance industries, animal care and rescue, funeral directors, alternative therapies and other entrepreneurs. My conclusions are based on 30 formal interviews, and reflections from many more informal conversations held during my teaching and counselling career. I am so grateful to the interviewees for their eagerness to be interviewed, and their honesty and vulnerability in the insights and experiences they shared. I was astonished by the similarity in the answers from the interviewees, regardless of their role, age and experience (The list of interviewees who were willing to be recognized can be found in the acknowledgement section at the back of the book).

The following statements summarize what I learned and the findings were consistent with all the interviewees regardless of profession or industry:

1. There was no mention of the need for personal well-being and the reminder to take care of themselves during any post-secondary education and training consistent across the sample.

2. They were not taught that burnout, compassion fatigue and PTSD could be a real possibility in their profession.

3. There is limited to no ongoing professional development that focuses on the need for personal well-being or education about compassion fatigue and PTSD. Since the completion of my interviews, a few social workers have shared that there has been a shift recently in providing education about self-care, compassion fatigue and burnout both in their programming and in the workplace.

INTRODUCTION: KEEPING IT TOGETHER?

4. They acknowledged they are encountering individuals affected by addiction and mental health issues in greater numbers and felt that education was lacking both in their training and on the job.

5. There was a lack of death and grief education for those who dealt with death and dying as part of their job. The information they were provided with was not current and it referred to how they could assist their clients and patients who were experiencing grief and not how they might manage it personally.

6. The stigma still exists when professionals seek mental health assistance and they confided that the available emotional support is often not helpful, as the providers lack the necessary skills to adequately support the specific needs of the individual.

7. Many professionals don't seek help because it suggests a vulnerability and an inability to do the job, and they definitely didn't feel safe confiding in their supervisor because it might impact their job placement and promotion and how they might be viewed by both their co-workers and supervisor.

8. First line workers identified a lack of empathy from supervisors and employers. Individuals were told they should have expected to be affected emotionally and physically and potentially be at risk for compassion fatigue and PTSD, given the career they chose.

9. The majority of them did not feel adequately prepared for their roles in the profession and found that it was on-the-job training that taught them the responsibilities of the job.

During the book writing process, I felt disheartened and at the same time hopeful—hopeful because in a world where we are constantly bombarded by distressing and heartbreaking news and given the rising emotional and physical cost to those in the helping professions, there are still many of us who seek positions to be of service to others.

I was disheartened when I became aware during my interview with Françoise Mathieu of the TEND Academy, which provides education and support around compassion fatigue and vicarious trauma, that she is now seeing individuals in careers we never thought would be affected by compassion fatigue, evidenced by the growing emotional distress. It seems more of us, regardless of profession, are now experiencing the effects of burnout and compassion fatigue, and therefore, it is even more important to focus on addressing the cause of our distress for our own health and the impact on our families, clients and friends.

Hope for the Future?

Our bodies are able to manage a great deal of physical stress; however, it's the emotional strain that takes its toll. Our bodies reflect our thoughts, and provide us with valuable information via a complex feedback system of emotions and symptoms. When we ignore these symptoms, we are at risk for disease, and a body out of rhythm reflects a life out of balance. I encourage you to read two wonderful books that elaborate further on the connection between our thoughts and emotions related to health conditions: *When the Body Says No* by Canadian physician Dr. Gabor Maté, and *You Can Heal Your Life* by Louise Hay.

INTRODUCTION: KEEPING IT TOGETHER?

It seems we have reached that point as predicted by Alvin Toffler whereby we aren't handling change and our emotions and society are suffering. Albert Einstein said, "Nothing happens until something moves," and, at this time with our lives out of balance, we are being urged to move now. The underlying premise of this book is to go boldly where we have not allowed ourselves to go before and put ourselves first. It's time we realized we deserve to flourish, not as a just reward for helping tirelessly or as a last resort when and if we have the time to listen to our heart's desire. Let's think about this differently and create a paradigm shift where it is accepted practice to value ourselves as much as we value those we help.

> Paraphrasing the message in Michael Jackson's song "The Man in the Mirror", if we want to make the world a better place it's time to look at ourselves and make a change while we have the time.

This book is a solution-focused guide filled with tools, resources and words of inspiration from authors that helped me. At the end of each chapter I have listed books and websites that I found beneficial, and I have also included a "playlist" of suggestions for further consideration and self-discovery. Just as one particular diet does not work for everyone, neither will some of the ideas and suggestions resonate with you. Take what you want and leave the rest. I have included as many quotes and stories from my interviewees as possible, and it is with regret that I was unable to use all their comments. Their love and positive energy was evident both in their willingness to participate in the project and in their intention to make a difference through sharing their experiences and insights.

Paraphrasing the message in Michael Jackson's song "The Man in the Mirror," if we want to make the world a better place it's time to look at ourselves and make a change while we have the time.

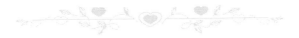

"You must make a choice to take a chance or your life will never change."

—ANONYMOUS

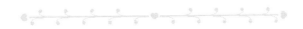

Inspiration and Wisdom of Others

Books

- *The Power of Intention* by Wayne Dyer
- *You Are a Badass: How to Stop Doubting Your Greatness and Start Living an Awesome Life* by Jen Sincero
- *The Compassion Fatigue Workbook: Creative Tools for Transforming Compassion Fatigue and Vicarious Traumatization* by Françoise Mathieu

Website

- www.tendacademy.ca—resources and training to address the complex needs of high-stress and trauma-exposed workplaces

PART ONE
Explore

"Above all we must realize that each of us makes a difference with our life. Each of us impacts the world around us every single day. We have a choice to use the gift of our life to make the world a better a place, or not to bother."

—JANE GOODALL

"What is necessary to change a person is to change his awareness of himself."

—ABRAHAM MASLOW

"Slow down and everything you are chasing will come around and catch you."

—JOHN DE PAOLA

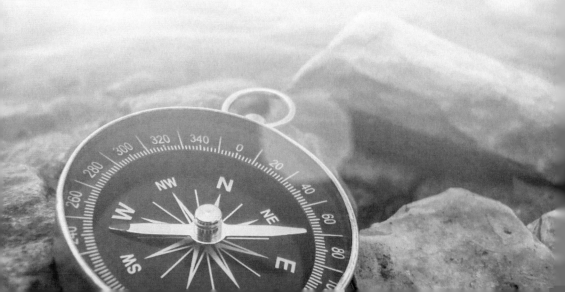

CHAPTER ONE

YOU GET WHAT YOU THINK ABOUT

We are the hurried and harried. There are numerous phrases that describe the frantic pace of our lifestyle: Hurry syndrome, time sickness and the disease of busyness, to name a few. Hurry syndrome is defined by online dictionaries as "a behaviour pattern characterized by continual rushing and anxiousness, an overwhelming and continual sense of urgency". It is further described as a "malaise in which a person feels chronically short of time and so tends to perform every task faster and gets flustered when encountering any kind of delay". Rapidly changing technology is designed to improve our lives and make things easier; however, often it does just the opposite. Data smog, a term coined by journalist David Shenk, refers to the overwhelming and voluminous amount of data and information that confuses us and makes it difficult to separate what is truthful or helpful. Our preoccupation with technology is another reason we can't seem to slow down and we continue on, at breakneck speed, living with the disease of busyness.

> "If we fill our newfound free time with more work, our technology has not freed us, but imprisoned us. More precisely, we have entrapped ourselves by becoming enamoured of machines at the expense of inner peace."
>
> —ALAN COHEN

We strive to be productive and efficient in both our professional and personal lives, and our measure of success relates to career and finance. We are numbers and data-driven. Unfortunately, the recurring refrain from the frontline social workers I interviewed was the pressure on them to perform with a focus on the number of clients "helped" and appropriate and complete documentation. How can there be a time limit on recovery as an indicator of the success for a counsellor working with a client? The time it takes to recover is contingent on the client's willingness and ability and the complexity of their issues and possible childhood trauma.

The counsellors I interviewed felt their supervisors didn't have an accurate perception of their workload and they didn't feel appreciated. In some of the organizations, there was no opportunity for support through clinical supervision as individuals in supervisory positions were unqualified to provide that supervision. I also heard from those in management positions that they genuinely wanted to be effective, support their staff and understand; however, many of them had no social work experience and were overwhelmed with the demands in a supervisory position. Without having done the job, how can managers and supervisors understand the plight of the frontline workers?

Meet Sandy Brooks, a social worker who left clinical work to become the Regional Implementation Coordinator for the Centre for Addiction and Mental Health. In this position, she focuses on building assets as she works with agencies to address their needs and then coaches them toward implementation using best practices. She chose to leave frontline work where she worked with overcoming deficits with her clients and this shifted her focus. She said the cost to her health was too great and her advice to other social workers is to know when to walk away: During our interview, she used the analogy of a filled-to-the-brim champagne flute to which you add baking soda, causing it to erupt over the top. She compared this to the amount of work and emotion you can handle and said when you have reached your limit and lost your buffer, you have the potential to erupt just like the champagne flute illustration. Sandy feels she is still helping but now is doing work, which, in her words, doesn't hurt her heart. She said when you have the gifts of listening, and engaging with those you serve and wanting to help, it hurts.

"Women in particular need to keep an eye on their physical and mental health, because if we're scurrying to and from appointments and errands, we don't have a lot of time to take care of ourselves. We need to do a better job of putting ourselves higher on our own 'to do' list."

—MICHELLE OBAMA

Women are encultured to be nurturers and look after others and they are showing the effects of this burden by the increasing number of physical conditions that previously were expressed more typically with men. In his book, *The Hurried Woman Syndrome*, gynaecologist Dr. Brent

Bost says that our busy lifestyle causes stress, and his book focuses on the effects of stress on women and states the hurried woman syndrome affects predominantly women between the age of 25 and 55 with children aged 4 to 16. The symptoms caused by hurry and stress are weight gain, low sex drive, moodiness and fatigue. I would suggest that the reason this age group of women are more susceptible is because they are doing too much: Likely working and perhaps carrying the majority of child care responsibilities in addition to potentially looking after parents as well. Women of all ages are also showing signs of other stress-related conditions such as hormonal imbalance, thyroid dysfunction, adrenal exhaustion and other physical and mental disorders.

Susan Bushell, EFT (emotional freedom technique) practitioner and instructor, who previously was a child and youth worker, used the term *female ghetto* in reference to those jobs that commonly have been held by women who earn less than men. If the amount of money one earns reflects your value and worth in society, then there is a belief that these jobs are less valuable, and by default so then are the individuals who do those jobs. The added drain on social worker's time and energy and others in social services results from duplicated services and/or family service based on multigenerational trauma. Susan described her female clients as looking haggard and tired, weighed down with the significant burdens of the job, and suggested there needs to be a unified movement by those professionals to provoke a much needed change.

> **Set your intention to focus on yourself and place your attention on what needs to shift.**

Many of my interviewees expressed concern that their jobs involve aspects of social work in addition to their own professional responsibilities. Marino Gazzola, retired staff sergeant with Guelph Police Department, said in our interview that young officers are now having to be social workers and that 50% of their calls are mental health interventions. "Mental health issues have risen 500–1000% over the past 10 years, and officers are seeing more complex problems now such as mental health issues, lack of resources, poverty and social problems with youth and kids." He said that young officers need more time with experienced officers due to the many facets of the job now.

Angela Spiller, RN, ONA Bargaining Unit President, also expressed similar concerns and informed me that more nurses are now employed in mental health facilities and retirement homes and face patients with dementia, leading to assaults, and they feel they lack the training and resources to do their jobs safely and effectively. "Nurses are frustrated with workload issues due to reduced funding that does not allow for appropriate staffing levels required to provide quality care. She says the inability to provide the best possible care to our patients results in job satisfaction, increased sick time related to both physical and psychological stresses." It seems that the need for social workers and training related to mental health concerns is growing, given our changing societal needs.

This chapter is about focusing on you and what's important to you. First, you need to slow down so you are aware of what you want and need. Set your intention to focus on yourself and place your attention on what needs to shift.

1. Be a Selfist

The term *selfist* means to be "for" ourselves. It's not selfish to do so and in fact it's necessary. By focusing on ourselves and our health (mind, body and spirit), we are healthier and our perspective shifts. Slowing down and disconnecting from the busyness of the world quiets the constant chattering of the ego, allowing us to access the wisdom of our intuition.

We create the space for much-needed awareness and guidance to surface, leading to change. Make the commitment to be a selfist and take the first step by purchasing a journal dedicated to self-discovery.

Ask yourself the following questions and don't censor your answers:

- If I had unlimited money, time and energy, how would I like to spend my time?
- What is preventing me from spending more time doing what I enjoy?
- What is missing from my life?
- What is one small step I could take to improve my life? Write it down, tell someone, schedule it.

"When you connect to the silence within you, that is when you can make sense of the disturbance going on around you."

—STEPHEN RICHARDS

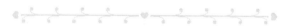

2. Make the Choice: Friendly or Hostile?

Albert Einstein stated that the most important question to ask is, do you believe you live in a hostile or a friendly universe? Your answer determines not only your perspective on life but also how you create your life, as your energy flows where your attention goes. Your life perspective affects your attitude and perception of your circumstances. We tend to label our stressors either as negative or positive. Events that we perceive as positive, such as a wedding or purchasing a house, can also cause us stress as we transition from being single to married or to being a homeowner. Stress is based on our perception of the situation, and when we worry excessively about something that may or may not happen, as in catastrophizing, we are thinking about something we don't want and emitting an energetic vibration of fear. If you believe the world is hostile, that it is out to get you and that illness and misfortune are lurking behind every corner, your thoughts and actions demonstrate that belief. Your attention will be on what is not going "right" in your life, and by declaring it good or bad, you emit a matching energetic signal.

> Remaining neutral removes your energy from the complaint, and focusing on what you can do results in more positive and empowered feelings.

You get what you think about whether you want it or not, according to Dr. Wayne Dyer. With the relentless flow of clients, it is not surprising that our enthusiasm and optimism perhaps give way to frustration with the system, and a growing sense of helplessness and hopelessness. Your thinking is focused on the problems, not the solutions, because there seem to be none. Pushing against something, resisting what is by protesting, judging and complaining, also adds energy to the issue. Remaining neutral removes your energy from the complaint, and focusing on what you can do results in more positive and empowered feelings.

If you watch the news, it's very difficult to believe in a world of good. I stopped watching the news many years ago because it negatively impacted my thoughts and I had difficulty maintaining a positive attitude. I challenge you to consider going news-free, for a day, a week and especially in the evening before bed. We program our subconscious mind with our thoughts before bed and when I watched the news, I found it difficult to remain positive and optimistic. The word *pronoia* was coined by astrologer Rob Brezsny, and means a belief in a world that is conspiring to shower us with blessings. Make the choice to not only believe in a friendly universe but also one that showers you with blessings.

Ask yourself:

Do I live in a hostile or friendly universe?

If you believe in a friendly universe, affirm daily, as often as possible: I live in a friendly and supportive universe. I am safe. All is well.

Note: An intention is a commitment to carrying out an action in the future. Some people like to state their intentions beginning with "I intend to…" This differs from an affirmation in that an affirmation is a declaration of something that is true or you want to be true. Affirmations are expressed in the present tense, use "I" as they are personal, and are positive. When setting intentions and using affirmations, they must resonate with what you believe, as it is emotion that ignites the statement with possibility

For example, if you do not have the mindset to state with confidence and believe you live in a friendly universe, use the affirmation: I am **open to believing in the possibility** that I live in a friendly universe. As your confidence, faith and trust increase, you could say, "I shift into believing…" Tailor your intentions and affirmations to align with what you believe.

3. Have an Attitude of Gratitude

Look for opportunities to be grateful. When you feel grateful, you elevate your consciousness to gratitude and you attract more to be grateful for through your energetic vibration. According to neuroscience, specifically the Hebbian theory, which proposes neurons that fire together wire together, you increase the likelihood that your attitude of gratitude and positive thinking becomes more prevalent.

Keep a gratitude list. Before going to sleep at night, pay attention to what you appreciated and were grateful for throughout the day.

4. Be Willing to Shift Your Perspective

Your thoughts and words are impressed upon your body and held in your body's tissues. Thoughts of stress and not coping will negatively affect your body, causing inflammation. Scientific research indicates that inflammation is the major cause of all chronic diseases. Be aware of your thoughts and the language you use when speaking about yourself and your circumstances. I challenge you to not only be "for" yourself but others as well. Don't engage in gossip and remove yourself from conversations that are about people who are not present.

When you disagree with what someone is saying, instead of reacting, respectfully say, "Thank you for your opinion," "Thank you for sharing," "Thank you for your thoughts on the subject," or "I never thought of it that way."

"You do not attract what you want, you attract what you are."

—WAYNE DYER

5. Be Relentlessly Solution-Focused (RSF)

Jason Selk, premier performance coach who works with athletes, coaches and business leaders developing mental toughness for high level success, suggests that you allow yourself just one minute to complain and focus on the problem. At the end of a minute, ask yourself, "What's the one thing I can do differently that would make this situation better?" This is a useful strategy, as it dramatically increases your chance at arriving at a solution, and any improvement, regardless how small, is still a shift toward focusing on a solution. RSF is characteristic of mental toughness, which Selk defines as "the ability to focus on and execute solutions, especially in the face of adversity". Practice RSF. Being solution-focused instead of problem-oriented results in a more positive perspective.

6. Simplify, Prioritize and Organize

Your actions indicate what you think is important. For example, you may value quality family time and connection, but not be present when your daughter is sharing about her day. How we spend our time reflects what we think is important and what we value. Be aware of how you spend your time each day.

Declutter your physical space and your weekly agenda. Prioritize what is important and consider what tasks you could let go of completely or delegate in your job and personal life. Helpers often have difficulty in delegating, so don't be surprised if you experience some resistance disguised as procrastination. When we declutter and prioritize, we feel more organized, and that feels good.

Ask yourself:

- Can I set aside some time as a family or couple or for myself and prioritize what is important and therefore schedule time in my day or week or month that reflects this commitment?
- Can I ask for help? Can I appreciate when I get the help I need and simply say "thank you"?
- More importantly, can I give what I need to myself? What do I need? Put it on the calendar.

7. Choose to Feel Good

Clement Stone suggested we make the choice to be an inverse paranoid and interpret everything as positive. Look for the good in every situation and person, and don't leave yourself out of this equation. Choose to feel good regardless of what's going on. Interpret everything you do with an attitude of appreciation and pride and learn to laugh at yourself when you make a mistake—it is through mistakes that we make corrections leading to success. I know of an organization that claps when someone makes a mistake, believing in the positive result through correction.

Affirm: "I believe in the perfect outcome to every situation in my life." Each morning before you get out of bed, set the intention to have a good day.

Ask yourself: What is it I must do today before the day is out to feel I had a good day? Intend to feel good no matter what.

8. Listen to Your Body

Many of us are used to relying on medical tests and procedures to determine our body's health; however, our body is communicating to us all the time and we need only to learn how to listen to the wisdom of our body. Intuitively, we know when something doesn't feel right and when we need to change our lifestyle choices and focus on our health. We need to make the shift to focusing on what health looks and feels like. Don't focus on what isn't working by listing a litany of complaints. Listen to what you say to others, family, patients and clients and what you hear them say to you. There is wisdom in those words, and the suggestions and advice you give to others could also be a message meant for you as well.

To support your health:

1. *Gather your health team.*

Build a team that supports you in perfect health (body, mind and spirit). Your team could consist of your doctor, naturopath, osteopath, counsellor and massage therapist. Be for yourself, and discuss your needs and concerns with the health-care practitioners who support you, respect your decisions and provide relevant and practical information so you can make informed choices about your health care while they work with you.

I was privileged to interview Luke Boudreau, Director of Operations for Chancellors Way Medical Arts Centre in Guelph. Luke confirmed what we all know—we can't take care of others if we don't take care of ourselves and don't take the time to make our health a priority. He believes we are pre-programmed for anxiety due in part to the instability of careers and jobs. Becky Beausaert is a sessional instructor at a number of local universities while waiting for a full-time position at just one university. She admits to being anxious and finds it a challenge to remain positive knowing tenure is difficult to secure when the trend is to hire less full-time contracts. This career instability affects her mood, sleep, her health and other lifestyle choices such as when would be the best time to begin a family. Becky finds participating in structured exercise a way to manage the stress while Luke meditates for 5- to 10-minute intervals during the day, and participates in sports such as power walking to better manage the demands on his time and energy.

Luke also talked about the shared community focus between the University of Guelph and the practitioners in their joint goal to address student concerns and also support for Guelph residents. The clinic is committed to efficiency and collaboration between all team members Walk with a Doc, which involves a 45-minute walk on a Saturday led by a doctor or other health practitioner from the clinic followed by social time at the clinic, is a program that encourages community building, wellness and a sense of belonging while walking and talking. For more information and to find a walk near you, visit www.walkwithadoc.org.

> As the obstacles surface on your path of change, which inevitably they will, remember they are the way. Rub your hands together and go for it with excitement and enthusiasm.

2. Detox and rejuvenate.

Seek to eliminate thoughts, food and substances that are toxic to your body and mind. Focus on building health within your body and be conscious of what you put in your body. Basically, hydrate, rest and move. In our culture, there is a certain amount of pride for those who sleep less and work more. According to Tom Rath, author of *Eat Move Sleep*, losing four hours of sleep is comparable to drinking a six pack of beer. He also says we show up to work even though we are sick with a cold, headache or too little sleep and although we are present, we are not performing at our best. He calls it "presenteeism".

We often don't drink enough water for optimal body function. Research is indicating that chronic disease is not just a result of aging but that dehydration over the years is also a contributing factor. I invite you to read Dr. Masaru Emoto's book *The Hidden Messages in Water*. Dr. Emoto discovered that crystals formed in frozen water reveal changes when specific, concentrated thoughts are directed towards them. This has implications about the use of our language on our own personal health due to our physical makeup and also our impact on the world.

The expression, "sitting is the new smoking" is gaining popularity and refers to the connection between less activity and increased health risks. Follow the 20–20 rule: 20 minutes of sitting and 20 seconds of movement. Be creative and find ways to increase activity during your day. For example, standing while on the phone, taking the stairs and sitting on an exercise ball instead of an office chair and bouncing slightly are all beneficial. Can you find the time to walk for 15 minutes a day, at the very least?

Ask yourself:

- What lifestyle choice can I make in support of my health?
- Can I commit to 28 days of this change so as to increase my chance of success in continuing this practice? Intend to commit to this choice by scheduling it on your calendar.
- Who needs to be part of my health team?

In conclusion of this chapter, I remind you of the choice to slow down. Sandy Brooks' advice in managing the frantic pace of life is to take the time to drink tea, together. Boiling the kettle, steeping the tea bag and drinking the cup is about slowing down and being present in the moment. As a frontline worker, she found it impossible to leave her work at the office and found counterbalancing the mental and emotional stress of her job with physical and social activity was helpful.

To help you move forward, focusing on what you want in the future, I have included a playlist. This is an opportunity to use your imagination and dream big while having fun.

Playlist

1. Before getting out of bed in the morning, focus on something that makes you feel good. Intend to have a good day.
2. Visualize your ideal life in all areas. Add as much detail as possible. Dream big. In the beginning, it was challenging to articulate exactly what I wanted in my life. I could only determine what I wanted in my life by reflecting on what I didn't want.
3. Based on your visualization, write out where you will be in one year from now. Be as specific as possible.

Inspiration and Wisdom of Others

Books

- *When the Body Says No* by Dr. Gabor Maté
- *You Can Heal Your Life* by Louise Hay
- *Manifest Your Destiny* by Wayne Dyer
- *The Universe Has Your Back* by Gabrielle Bernstein
- *The Hidden Messages in Water* by Masaru Emoto

Websites

- www.thethyroidpharmacist.com—connection between stress, the thyroid, hormones and weight gain
- www.heatherkjones.com—dietitian who focuses on the mind-body connection
- www.calmlifestylemedicine.ca
- www.walkwithadoc.org
- www.luckybitch.com—overcoming self-limiting beliefs around money
- www.findperspective.org—real-life stories about people who uplift and inspire
- www.spiritjunkie.com

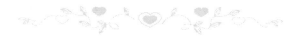

"You, yourself, as much as anybody in the entire universe, deserve your love and affection."

—BUDDHA

Pour some tea,

settle in

and turn the page.

"We all know that the feminine values of well-being, love, connection, inclusion and caring are critical to creating a world that works. But what if these feminine values are the keys to creating the life of your dreams?"
—KRIS CARR

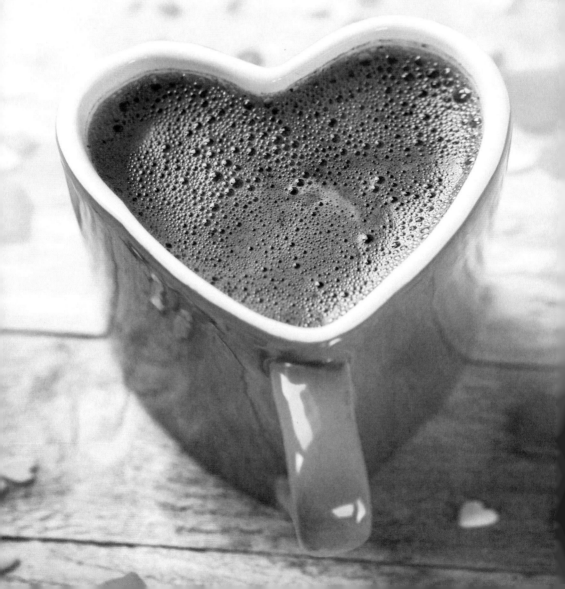

CHAPTER TWO

LOVE IS AN ACTION WORD

The previous chapter encouraged you to commit to focusing on yourself as a selfist. This chapter is about courage; the root word for courage is "coeur", meaning heart. The heart is associated with courage, love, compassion, wisdom and strength. We all desire to love and be loved, and that's not for the faint of heart.

Love opens us up and expands our thinking and therefore our lives, while fear causes us to shrink and contract. When we believe we live in a hostile universe, our actions are motivated by fear and we feel scared, anxious and tense. Fear also prevents us from being in the flow, just like a kinked garden hose that obstructs the flow of water. This inflexible thinking can also be expressed in our body as stiffness in our joints and we don't move with ease. When we are motivated by love, our world reflects that belief and our life flows. Love is an action word.

"Your heart is the light of this world; don't cover it with your mind."

—MOOJI

1. Love Yourself

It feels good to help; however, those actions should not define who we are. We are beings, not doings, or doers. When we focus on extending our love to ourselves first and then to others and make that our reason for working with others, they feel that shift in our energy. We can raise them up by raising our vibration to that of love.

The following is a list of traits associated with helpers. These traits could explain why we may be resistant to admitting we love ourselves and taking actions that demonstrate self-love in addition to taking care of ourselves and what we need.

How many of these traits describe you? There is no judgment, shame or blame in this; it's an awareness tool. Being aware is the first step to change.

Traits of Helpers:

1. How you feel about yourself is based on what you do and how well you do it.
2. You thrive on fixing problems and you are very productive.
3. You are much better at giving than receiving, and you have difficulty delegating and asking for help and support.
4. You are an idealist and have difficulty acknowledging mistakes and limitations because they suggest vulnerability, weakness and failure.
5. Practicing self-care is a challenge.

"I have an everyday religion that works for me. Love yourself first and everything else falls into place."

—LUCILLE BALL

Do you have the courage to admit you love and accept yourself as you are? Your self-concept and self-confidence depend on it. It doesn't mean you can't aspire to improve; however, how you feel about yourself determines your value, monetary and otherwise. When my children were growing up, I had a piece of paper on the front door with the words: "I love, accept and appreciate you." Every time my children left the house, they read this message, and they knew they could be themselves and that they were loved for who they were, not what they did. As a family each week we chose to focus on a virtue from *The Family Virtues Guide: Simple Ways to Bring Out the Best in Our Children and Ourselves* by Linda Kavelin-Popov. I also used the companion guide *Virtues Project Educators Guide: Simple Ways to Create a Culture of Character* in my classroom.

> Can you look in the mirror and say, "I love, accept and appreciate you?"

Can you look in the mirror and say, "I love, accept and appreciate you?" If you find that a challenge, you might be more comfortable with "I like you". Do you have the courage to look in the mirror and say this every day for the next 30 days? Your life will change using this one strategy.

Balance is about valuing and helping ourselves as much as we value and help others. Counsellor Elizabeth Kupferman says caretaking is rooted in insecurity and a need to be in control and is a trait of co-dependency, while caregiving is an expression of kindness. She believes these two exist on a continuum, and that we can't be a caretaker and a caregiver at the same time. As helpers, we should be aware where our tendencies lie and aim to practice more caregiving traits than caretaking. Where do you fit on Elizabeth Kupferman's continuum found below? The complete continuum can be found at www.soberrecovery.com. I also refer you to the book *When Society Becomes an Addict* by Anne Wilson Schaef, and Melody Beattie's books for more useful information on co-dependency.

Caretaking feels stressful, exhausting and frustrating. Caregiving feels right and feels like love. It reenergizes and inspires you.

Caretaking crosses boundaries. Caregiving honours them. Caretakers don't practice self-care because they mistakenly believe it is a selfish act.

Caregivers practice self-care unabashedly because they know that keeping themselves happy enables them to be of service to others.

Caretakers worry; caregivers take action and solve problems. Caretakers think they know what's best for others; caregivers only know what's best for themselves.

Caretaking creates anxiety and/or depression in the caretaker. Caregiving decreases anxiety and/or depression in the caregiver.

Caretakers start fixing when a problem arises for someone else; caregivers empathize fully, letting the other person know they are not alone and lovingly asks "What are you going to do about that?"

> "The number one relationship that determines the quality of all the others in your life and sets the tone for them, is the one you have with yourself."
>
> —CHRISTIANE NORTHRUP

2. Choose Love, Not Fear

There's a Native American story that illustrates the choice we must make between love and fear. One day, a grandfather was talking to his grandson and told him there are two wolves inside each of us and they're always at war. One wolf represents love, kindness and bravery, while the other wolf represents fear, greed and hatred. The grandson thinks for a moment and asks his grandfather which wolf wins and his grandfather replied, "The one you feed."

"Love is what we are born with. Fear is what we learn. The spiritual journey is the unlearning of fear and prejudices and the acceptance of love back in our hearts. Love is the essential reality and our purpose on earth. To be consciously aware of it, to experience love in ourselves and others, is the meaning of life. Meaning does not lie in things. Meaning lies in us."

—MARIANNE WILLIAMSON

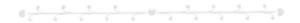

We have a choice in every moment to place our attention on either love or fear. As Marianne Williamson's quote states, fear is what we have learned, and it takes commitment to choose to believe in a world that's positive and choose love as often as possible. While in teachers' college, we watched the film "Cipher in the Snow", and the message in the movie later became my teaching philosophy. The movie is about a young boy who nobody paid attention to and it is not until he dies that the community and school take the time to discover who he is. They uncover his troubled family life and then are full of regret that they didn't take the time to get to know him. During my teaching career, I made a point of greeting my students at the door, addressing them by name and speaking to as many of them as possible over the course of the day. I wanted them to know their presence in my class was important to me and that I cared. I hoped that if they needed my help, they would feel comfortable enough to reach out.

In his book, *The Divine Matrix,* Gregg Braden identifies three universal fears, and believing in any one of them makes it a challenge to live from your heart. Feelings of inadequacy trigger the belief in the first fear: Low self-worth. We compare ourselves to others, judge ourselves more harshly than anyone else and believe we are not enough. If you resonate with this fear, you are not alone. Bestselling author, speaker and therapist Marisa Peer says the biggest disease facing humanity is "I am not enough." She says we crave praise from those who are closest to us and when it doesn't happen, we misinterpret that as we are not enough. From that point on, we struggle with feeling good about ourselves. I encourage you to watch her 40-minute talk on YouTube called, *The Biggest Disease Affecting Humanity: "I'm Not Enough"*. It is engaging and enlightening.

The second fear identified by Gregg is the fear of trusting and surrendering. This is about letting go the need to control and fix, and having faith. Having faith means trusting it will work out and being open to a solution. Marianne Williamson says, "Faith isn't blind; it is visionary. Having faith in a positive outcome doesn't mean you're denying a problem or ignoring obstacles; it simply means you are affirming a solution." This reinforces the idea of inverse paranoia and the expectation of a positive outcome. Life flows when we choose love, while fear results in constriction and a life of struggle and suffering.

> We have a choice in every moment to place our attention on either love or fear.

The fear of separation and abandonment is the third fear Gregg identifies. He suggests the underlying reason for this fear is our separation from our higher power and the belief that we are alone and have to do everything ourselves. We are triggered whenever anyone leaves us. For example, if our parents divorce when we are young and we don't see one parent regularly, when we are older, we are triggered when relationships break up and also when people don't listen and pay attention to us.

The imagery that helps me maintain faith and trust in the support of the universe, or in a power greater than me, is courtesy of Wayne Dyer. Imagine riding a tram or train and there's a strap suspended overhead to hang on to for support. Dyer encourages us to reach overhead for the strap whenever we are in need of guidance, allowing our "senior partner," his words, to be in charge. The expression "Let go and let God" emphasizes the same idea. All three fears are in relationship to and with each other and we often find we are subject to triggers involving a belief in one, two or three of them.

"Whenever you meet anyone, remember they are going through a great war."

—RALPH WALDO EMERSON

3. Live from the Heart

There is little awareness about the power of the heart relative to how much we know about the brain. Did you know that the heart's electromagnetic field extends several feet from your body, changes with your emotions and communicates with the brain, sending more information to the brain than the brain sends to it? When we're in close proximity with people, they sense our energetic vibration and are affected by our heart's electromagnetic field as it extends outward from our body, and we are also affected by theirs. When we focus on extending our love to others, consciously extending our heart field, they feel that shift in energy. We not only raise our vibration; we raise theirs as well.

Living from the heart means demonstrating the qualities of compassion, love, wisdom, courage and strength, and emphasizes feeling and thinking when you make a decision. There's an expression from *A Course in Miracles*, "Everything is either an expression of love or a call for love". Remembering those words has helped me in my relationships at home, work and with my clients. When I encounter a person who is triggering a reaction in me and I make the choice to switch off the automatic, conditioned reaction by pausing and breathing, I am able to respond rather than react. I focus on seeing the good in them and the situation and extending love. Our words and actions, from love, with love, make a difference to everyone we meet.

> Living from the heart means demonstrating the qualities of compassion, love, wisdom, courage and strength, and emphasizes feeling and thinking when you make a decision.

Can you, in an emotional situation, pause and see the situation as either love or a cry for love and respond rather than react?

"Work is love made visible."

—KAHLIL GIBRAN

4. Love What You Do

Meet Kelly Romanick, Moksha Yoga studio owner and massage therapist. I loved what she said about her work: "When you are engulfed in your passion it's like you are in love. You are in the flow and not aware of your energy output so you need people around you to remind you of that." She said, if you have a push at work, it is up to you to schedule a more modest week in the near future. It takes discipline, she said, to be well. You need to plan downtime. Decide what you want your day to look like with the goal of feeling good. Experiment and if you can't do what you planned or it doesn't feel good, then rethink your plan.

Intend to feel good at work with the focus on remaining positive. Play to your strengths as much as possible for as much of your day as possible, and boost your self-confidence and enjoyment. If you don't love what you do, find some aspect of your job you do love and concentrate on that. When I struggle with maintaining a positive attitude and feeling good, I strive to reach for a better feeling emotion. In the book *Ask and It Is Given* by Abraham Hicks, they suggest a scale of emotions beginning with the lowest vibrational emotion, shame. I use this scale to "upscale" my emotions incrementally when I find myself in a challenging situation, as that is more doable when I'm struggling with extending love.

5. Teach People How to Treat You

We teach people how to treat us by our words and actions. Your feelings, wants and needs are important, and you may need to say "no" to honour what you want and need. As interdependent beings, when we take care of ourselves by saying "no," it encourages others to do the same. Use your words to let people know what you're feeling, what you want and need and encourage them to also use their words to articulate what they want and need. You have a right to say "no" and for some of us this requires practice as we have often put other people's needs and happiness before our own, believing we are responsible for their feelings. We have no control over how others feel nor is it our responsibility. We are responsible for articulating what we need and want and making people aware of our boundaries by our words and actions. Practice saying "no".

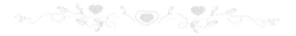

"First and foremost, if we maintain healthy emotional boundaries and direct love and kindness inwards, we are taking care of ourselves, and, secondly, we are giving a subliminal message to others about how we wish to be treated. People tend to subconsciously treat us how we treat ourselves."

—CHRISTOPHER DINES

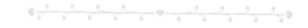

6. Be Real

We are feeling beings, and emotion is simply energy in motion. Stuffing our emotions or pressing down our feelings to avoid pain can result in disease and depression. What we resist persists, and our body will communicate the need to express our feelings with symptoms and conditions. Some of us might believe that in the role we play, it isn't appropriate to express our emotions. More often than not, it increases people's level of comfort with us when we do let our guard down and "be real".

Ponder this: Where in your body do you hold your emotions? Where do you need to direct your attention based on what your body is telling you?

7. To Love Is to Grieve

The depth that we feel grief over a loss is proportionate to the depth of feelings we had for the person who died. We grieve for clients and patients who have died and we also experience the death of pets, family members and suffer other losses, not just related to the physical death of someone or something. Transition or change not related to a physical death is also accompanied by feelings of loss. It's okay to feel sad. It's a natural response to the loss of something or someone we cared about. It's in our best interest to feel our feelings rather than to stuff them and to that end I believe we need grief and death education for us first most importantly and then as it relates to our clients and how we can best take care of them.

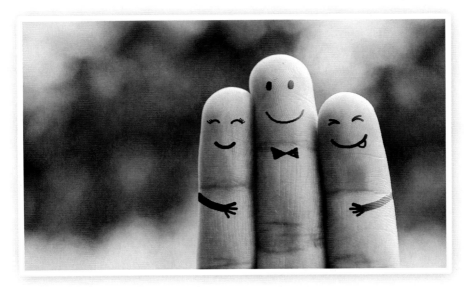

The following excerpt eloquently describes the loss and grief related to our jobs. Regrettably, I have lost the reference and whom to credit these beautifully written words. I am very appreciative and grateful to the author:

"We have all lost our innocence once we entered into our chosen profession. We grieve for the loss of our dreams, the fact we can't seem to make it better for others that we don't seem to be making a difference. And we are definitely affected by the sadness we hear and witness in those human beings we work with. Their stories stir up our compassion and speak to our hearts. The very reasons we are good at our jobs, as in empathy, sensitivity and compassion, are also the reasons why we are moved to tears and feel sad. Out of a need to survive and continue day to day, hearing and seeing more, we stuff these feelings, resisting the tears, believing we will get used to this, that if we don't open that door, we can escape that emotion. Eventually we are so turned off, out of a need to do our jobs, and our grief surfaces in other ways. Irritability, intolerance and apathy are some of the many faces of grief."

"Sorrow is an inseparable dimension of our human experience. We suffer a loss because we are human. And in our suffering, we are transformed."

—ALAN WOLFELT

I consider Alan Wolfelt the expert for information and support related to death, grief and mourning. I would encourage you to visit his website for support and education. I was introduced to Alan's work at a free workshop for professionals held at Bay Gardens Funeral Home in Hamilton, and I was impressed by their commitment to public education and conducting workshops for professionals as they're addressing a need for both. I admire their dedication to that mission and interviewed two of their funeral directors, Lynne Atkinson and Amy McCartney. They shared that people who pursue a career in the funeral industry believe it is a calling and are empathetic, and compassionate and very likely have experienced grief associated with death. They agreed that it certainly isn't for everyone, and that they both chose this work because they cared and wanted to help not because of the money as an existing stereotype suggests.

Both Lynne and Amy would like to see a course that supports funeral directors and their grief. They felt education around grief and death was missing in their training and in continuing education.

Erin McInnis is also passionate about creating opportunities for discussions related to death. She's a social worker employed as the Community Service Coordinator at Hospice Wellington. In our interview, she also mentioned the ritual of tea drinking, and elaborated further stating that in her experience 95% of the time, people just need someone to talk to, not necessarily needing a trained counsellor. Erin was drawn to this work in part due to the death of her mom when she was 16, and her philosophy is not "if" but "when" which led to her interest in death education. She initiated Death Cafés in Guelph, and to date has held six cafés, to which 200 people have attended. She encourages others to join the global movement and create their own death café. Please check out the website and guidelines to open the conversation in your community.

Ponder this: Would you consider increasing your comfort level with death, grief and mourning by attending a workshop or death café? If so, make the commitment and find a workshop that appeals to you.

Am I willing to confront my own emotions around deaths in my experience with a friend or professional?

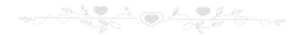

"We burn out not because we don't care but because we don't grieve. We burn out because we've allowed our hearts to become so filled with loss that we have no room left to care."

—DR. RACHEL REMEN

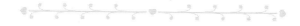

8. Love Life Just the Way It Is

The definition of *joie de vivre* is a feeling of happiness or excitement about life. Accept who you are, accept others and what's going on in the world and by this statement I'm not suggesting we don't care about what's happening in the world. I encourage you to focus on what's going right in the world and don't focus on and add your energy to causes and activities that aren't in alignment with love. Choose love and hold your energy in that vibration rather than in fear and anger. Make choices that honour your heart and are meaningful to you. Do what you love each day and live with the rhythm of the heart. Treat yourself to something you love and spend time with people you love.

Playlist

1. Love yourself enough to… Is there something that needs your attention? Feel the fear and do it anyway.
2. Answer these three questions: What do you love about yourself? What are you good at? What do you love to do? Seek opportunities to express this love.
3. Is there an organization or job that could benefit from what you have to offer? Take inspired action. Inspired action is taking a step towards change that scares and excites you.

Inspiration and Wisdom of Others

Books

- *The Divine Matrix* by Gregg Braden
- *Return to Love* to Marianne Williamson
- *Goddesses Never Age* by Christiane Northrup
- *Women's Bodies, Women's Wisdom* by Christiane Northrup

Websites

- www.heartmath.com
- www.marisapeer.com
- www.centerforloss.com (Alan Wolfelt)
- www.hospicewellington.org
- www.thecopingcentre.com

"Not all of us can do great things. But we can do small things with great love."

—MOTHER THERESA

Love yourself

enough to turn the page.

"Owning our own story can be hard but not nearly as difficult as spending our lives running from it."
—BRENÉ BROWN

"Our stories hold unique inspiration for one another."
—LAILAH GIFTY AKITA

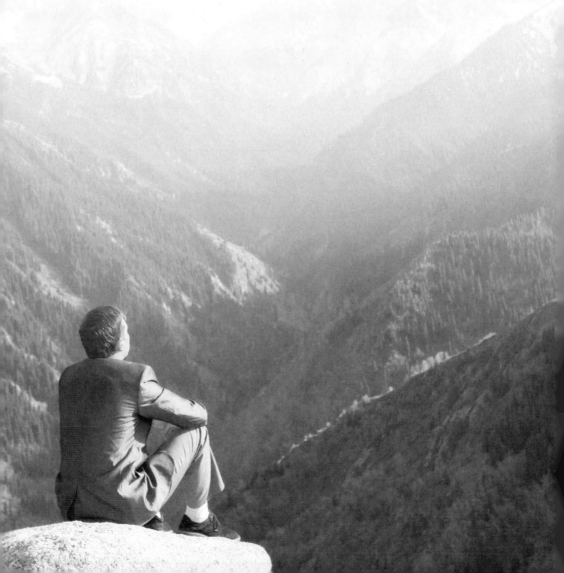

CHAPTER THREE

STUCK IN A RUT, OR ARE YOU?

Being willing to look at the stories of our lives and unravel the tapestry of experiences that have made us who we are today takes courage. Very few of us are eager to be vulnerable enough to feel and process the pain of our experiences. We resist the opportunity by ignoring, denying and distracting ourselves by life and helping others. When we refuse to look at and own our stuff, we will be triggered when others share and then we aren't as helpful as a result.

The word vulnerability is derived from the Latin *vulnus*, wound, and suggests the potential for humans to be wounded both physically and psychologically. Many of us pursued our careers because we felt a calling based on a hurt we experienced. The term *wounded healer* recognizes that the expertise and insights we gained from our experiences are helpful to others in similar circumstances. Embedded in the emotionally painful situations of adversity is the experience to draw forth our inner strength and body wisdom by being present to the lesson, reframing the story and finally accepting and embracing the personal growth opportunity.

> "Vulnerability is not weakness. And that myth is profoundly dangerous. Vulnerability is the birthplace of innovation, creativity and change."
>
> —BRENÉ BROWN

Author of the book *The Human Magnet Syndrome: Why We Love People Who Hurt Us* and practicing psychotherapist Ross Rosenberg believes that helping professionals need to practice what they preach. He believes that it if we take care of our own emotional issues, we develop more compassion, understanding and empathy while increasing awareness and understanding of our own feelings of vulnerability, anxiety or fear. He also believes that we are negligent if we don't take care of our health because of the role we play. From this mindset, he created the Golden Rule for the Helping Professionals and you can find the complete list and background information on the website: www.selfgrowth.com.

> Embedded in the emotionally painful situations of adversity is the experience to draw forth our inner strength and body wisdom by being present to the lesson, reframing the story and finally accepting and embracing the personal growth opportunity.

1. Commit to Dealing with Your Stuff

To be as helpful as possible in our role, there's a need to look at our own stuff, first and foremost for our own health and also as a role model for our clients, co-workers and children. We look at where we are unhealed, and know that shadow side we are ashamed of is where transformation could result if we were brave enough to own that part of us. We claim our personal power through responsibility, and with a sense of acceptance and discrement. We take what we want and leave the rest.

2. Give Up the Drama

This, too, shall pass. This is one of my favourite expressions. Whether you are in a situation that you interpret as positive or negative, the circumstance is temporary, so there is no need to get wrapped up in the drama at the time. When we decide to make a change and focus on ourselves, sometimes, even though we wanted out of the drama, trauma and the chaos, we are uncomfortable with the peace and time to spend on ourselves. It scares us. Breathe and make the choice to look forward and take an inspired step, even ever so small. Whatever situation you find yourself, this, too, shall pass.

3. Make Friends with Your Shadow

Everything that triggers us is either a mirror to see ourselves more clearly or a projection. We either like what we see or we blame others because we have projected our own dislike of self onto someone else. We judge in others what we cannot accept about ourselves. There is always something to learn through facing an obstacle; we just may not "get it" at first.

Meet Leanne Giavedoni. She is a physiotherapist who left her position in a hospital to become a wellness coach with the intention to "help the helpers", and she created Mindful Physio. During our interview Leanne said struggle is your greatest gift. It 's your shadow work and you can truly help people because of the experience you have had. She says the situation doesn't necessarily change; it is our perspective that shifts and so we are different.

4. Let Go of Expectations

You are not in charge of someone else's choices or health. When we see others struggling (clients, friends and family), it's difficult not to want or try to fix things for them. Andrea Farrell, a paramedic, identified a steep learning curve when she first started in her profession. People refused treatment, and she had to be okay with that as their choice. She found that a challenge as were some of the daily "routine" calls. One of her most emotional calls was arriving to transport a 40-year-old palliative patient to hospice and witnessing her say goodbye to her dog for the last time. Andrea also identified the lack of information follow-up to paramedics about the health condition of those they transport. Within a few months, they do receive a brief description of the outcome and general health details, gender and age of the patient, but no name. The time lag has blurred the event, and she finds it difficult to remember the patient. While she is grateful for some information she wishes for improvements in that communication in addition to greater opportunities for professional support.

5. Let Yourself off the Hook

We must be willing to invest in ourselves: Our health, physically, mentally and emotionally to be available to others. Some of us are responsible for others in life and death situations and have been taught to "have saves" like in firefighting. Brad Enright, fire captain, chose to become a captain to look after other firefighters having experienced PTSD as a result of the emotional cost of the job. He told me that he hadn't known he was suffering until he went into counselling for another reason. He could not stress enough the need for qualified counsellors to avoid re-traumatizing in legitimizing the injury as a problem. His advice to new firefighters is "No matter what you think, this job is going to hurt you—physically, mentally and emotionally—while if you get to an incident and it doesn't, then you have other issues. Don't pretend you are strong and it doesn't hurt as that will cause problems. Seek help."

Both Brad and Marino, in their supervisory roles, are committed to helping the firefighters and officers who report to them because they've done the job and are able to subtly suggest when help is needed, recognizing the potential for emotional and physical injury. There still exists a stigma among first responders who use language like the "kiss and hug brigade", suggesting it is not accepted to seek support in response to the inherent emotion of the job. Perhaps in time this stigma will lessen when we accept that these jobs result in emotional trauma, and therefore it's a necessary precaution to guard against burnout, compassion fatigue and PTSD and maintaining personal well-being.

Is it possible that within the expectation of "having saves" there could be room for a reality check? Can first responders, even though they do their best, recognize some situations were impossible? Can you let yourself off the hook knowing you did the best job you could? I specifically make reference to firefighters and police personnel in this section, however I use the term first responders to include all those helpers who are involved in physical trauma scenes. This involves medical staff, paramedics and emergency services firefighters, police personnel, soldiers, victim services and in large scale trauma also involves counsellors and other support services. My apologies if I have excluded any other helpers, it has not been intentional in any way.

I am so grateful for all these helpers who willingly pursue this work dealing with trauma, injury and death daily. By suggesting the possibility of acceptance and forgiveness it is not my intention to devalue the huge responsibility of the job, and without doing the job I realize I can't possibly know what it feels like to experience the emotional weight of that responsibility. I hope that we can arrive at a place where first responders feel valued for the job they do, and that they recognize a job with such a high price requires emotional and physical support and they feel accepted in seeking that support without fear of judgement.

Processing through debriefing with a trained professional and perhaps also with a caring partner, either spouse or co-worker is helpful and necessary. We haven't been taught this, so it will only happen if we have the intention to do it. Hopefully, through counselling and expressing feelings, in time the pain is lessened and leads to compassion, acceptance and forgiveness of self, a salve to your soul.

Many of the individuals I spoke to identified the importance of having the support of their partner; however, they were cautious about disclosing details so as not to traumatize their partners.

"To see your drama clearly is to be liberated from it."

—KEN KEYES JR.

6. Just Do It

I encourage you to explore the experiences within your unique life story, seeing them as opportunities that transform and eventually leading to a life that is flourishing because of those challenges. Remember, you are not your story. The following process comes from B Grace Bullock, PhD, *Mindful Relationships – Seven Skills for Success: Integrating the Science of Mind, Body and Brain.*

Take a few moments to write down your personal identity story. You may use simple descriptive phrases like "I am tough," "I take care of others before myself," and "I am good at math." You may also choose to write down experiences, family beliefs or other influences that helped to shape how you view yourself now. Once you have listed your beliefs about yourself, and identified a few of your stories, look at each one and ask yourself the following questions:

1. Where did this story come from?
2. Is this my story or someone else's?
3. Is this story true of me now?
4. Is this story contributing to or undermining my happiness?
5. Do I choose to continue to live this story or is it time to write a new one?

"No birthing of anything new can occur without the dying of the old."
—MARIANNE WILLIAMSON

I use another process with my clients that I created called Your Timeline Life Review:

1. Look back over your life and highlight significant events.
2. Write out scenarios, or use short phrases to remind you of those experience in a chart
3. Some clients have documented their life circumstances on a line graph with appropriate dips and rises based on the emotion of the event.
3. Are there are any trends in behaviour, in thoughts and even situations? Are there common themes?
4. Is there any remaining emotion that still needs to be processed? And, most importantly, how does this inform where you are now?
5. What do you need to do to improve your life by applying what you have learned?

7. What is the Silver Lining? Celebrate

During the timeline life review, focus on your successes, your triumphs. At first glance, you can see the obvious "happy" experiences and what learning you gained. Over time and with some processing and reflection with a counsellor, or in your journal, with a safe caring friend or partner, you will be able to identify the events you once perceived as negative and celebrate what you learned through that experience as well. You owned your story and took the time to uncover the gift within the experience and you are still standing. In fact, you are standing in your power. Celebrate that victory!

8. Forgive Yourself

I used to think one day I would arrive, as in be finished with my life lessons, having done all my inner work; however, I know now that the work is never done. In processing our life stories, we can feel some regret or shame, however, it is in our best interest to let those feelings go and forgive ourselves. From there we can forgive others with the understanding that it takes two for a relationship to fail, or be successful. We both have a part to play.

Forgiving someone is not condoning and accepting the behaviour. I suggest that forgiveness is giving for ourselves, and letting ourselves off the hook of suffering. Holding on to those feelings is like drinking poison and expecting the other person to die. Think of forgiveness as selective remembering, and focus on remembering the love you experienced within the painful circumstance. Once you focus on the positive and forgive the situation, you are free. I have found Colin Tipping's work on forgiveness to be helpful, and his book is listed in the resource section at the end of the chapter.

I also suggest considering the Hawaiian process, Ho'oponopono as a way to process and let go of painful experiences. I urge you to Google search Dr. Len, and read about his life-changing work with inmates at a psychiatric prison. He is the creator of the Ho'oponopono process that uses four simple statements, one of which is "Please forgive me." When I have been challenged with forgiving an individual I have used this process and it reduced the energetic vibration of anger finally leading to forgiveness. I also have used the expression "I am willing to forgive this person…" as an intermediary step. Forgiveness is a process. Recognize that, be gentle with yourself and don't "should" on yourself expecting you have to forgive someone. That is a personal choice and dependent on the inflicted injury.

Trauma and Adverse Childhood Experiences

I was introduced to the Adverse Childhood Experience (ACE) study about 10 years ago, and it changed how I viewed the students and teachers I worked with. The study concluded that people who had difficult or adverse experiences (e.g., stress, divorce, trauma and abuse) in childhood were at greater risk of both physical and mental health problems during adulthood. The ACE study did not include resiliency factors that might be present in a child's life, just the adverse conditions. I found this study helpful because it reminded me to be compassionate with all, as you never know someone's personal history. I am thrilled that there are schools in the States that use the ACE study and am hopeful that Canada will follow suit. I believe we all need to be trauma-aware and sensitive, especially if we work with young people so we don't unconsciously re-wound a child with our comments or actions. Françoise Mathieu believes we should all be trauma informed, especially those in law enforcement, primary care physicians and those in the justice system. As a society, we would be gentler and more compassionate.

I had the pleasure of interviewing Brad Enright, the firefighter mentioned earlier in this chapter. He suffered from PTSD, undiagnosed for months by counsellors available through his job's benefits. Brad managed okay or so he thought, until the ongoing emotionality of his job began to add up and compound an already difficult childhood and recent marital issues. It wasn't until he attended couples' counselling with his wife in a last-ditch attempt to save his marriage that the counsellor asked him if he had considered that he might be suffering from PTSD. In an open and honest dialogue with me he shared significant events from his childhood and as a young parent. He questioned whether if he had appropriate support earlier, perhaps the severity of his own mental health wouldn't have been so significant, and the job impact not have had such significant ramifications. After a year of therapy, he is said he is in a more positive place, his marriage repaired and thriving, along with his relationships with his children.

Kilbride and Associates facilitate trauma education workshops for interested organizations and school boards. A comprehensive list of their services can be found at the end of the book.

Playlist

I encourage you to explore the experiences within your unique life story, seeing them as opportunities that transform and eventually leading to a life that is flourishing because of those challenges.

1. Make a commitment to dealing with your stuff. Choose one method and go for it. Suggestions are: by Byron Katie, *Radical Forgiveness* by Colin Tipping or *Timeline Life Review*. There are free worksheets and resources on both Byron's and Colin's websites. Remember, you don't need to do this alone. Seek support from a professional, a counsellor with or without assistance from

an energy practitioner. Emotional Freedom Technique (EFT) is very helpful in releasing the energy associated with the emotion of an event. I have included EFT contacts in the resource section.

2. Counterbalance the emotional and mental with social and physical. This chapter has likely been challenging, so find something fun to do, and commit to it by putting it on the calendar.

3. Visualize challenging experiences from your past having the outcome you would have liked. This is another way of changing your story which leads to feelings of empowerment and positivity.

4. Take care of yourself. What does that look like? What do you need? Don't hesitate to seek the support you need.

Inspiration and Wisdom of Others

Books

- *Loving What Is: Four Questions That Can Change Your Life* by Byron Katie
- *In the Realm of Hungry Ghosts: Close Encounters with Addiction* by Dr. Gabor Maté
- *Scattered Minds: A New Look at the Origins and Healing of Attention Deficit Disorder* by Dr. Gabor Maté
- *Daring Greatly: How the Courage to Be Vulnerable Transforms the Way We Live, Love, Parent, and Lead* by Brené Brown
- *Radical Forgiveness: Making Room for the Miracle* by Colin Tipping
- *The Human Magnet Syndrome: Why We Love People Who Hurt Us* by Ross Rosenberg

Websites

- www.melodybeattie.com—co-dependency, recovery, grief, abuse, meditation and support
- www.thework.com
- www.drgabormate.com
- www.acestudy.org
- www.radicalforgiveness.com
- www.lorettalaroche.com—humour
- www.freeyouremotions.com—Susan Bushell, EFT instructor and practitioner
- www.emofree.com

Supportive Communities

- AA, NA, Al Anon, etc.
- Unity Church for Practical Christianity, Kitchener or www.unity.org
- Homewood Health Centre, Guelph

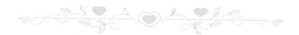

*"Let's forgive the past and who we were then.
Let's embrace the present and who we're capable of becoming.
Let's surrender the future and watch miracles unfold."*

—MARIANNE WILLIAMSON

Raise your hands up in the air in celebration.

With excitement and anticipation, turn the page.

PART TWO
Transform

"Flock with others who are truly, madly and deeply in love with life."

—IAN LAWTON

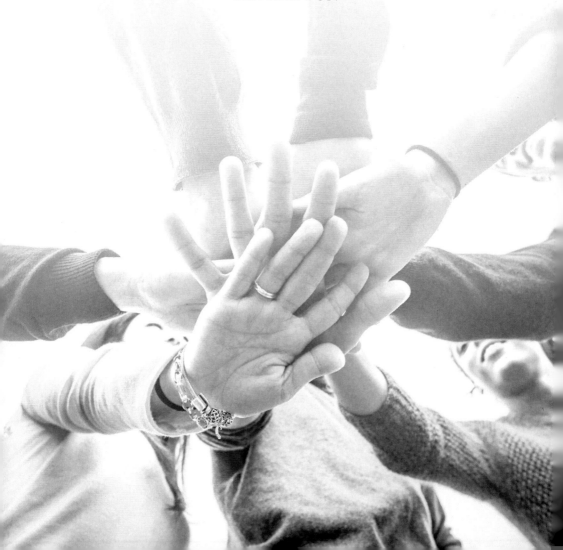

CHAPTER FOUR

DANCING AS FAST AS I CAN

You are not alone in the busyness of your life, although the speed of life often makes you feel like you are rushing and isolated from others. Researchers found that the happiest people are those that have a tribe, and that isolation and loneliness contribute to major health risks.

The Roseto effect describes how a close-knit Italian community in Pennsylvania escaped the risk of heart attacks despite having unhealthy lifestyles. In 1960, Dr. Stephen Wolf conducted a study of the socially isolated community of Roseto, Pennsylvania. He found that no one under the age of 55 died of a heart attack, and the death rate from heart attacks for men over the age of 65 was half the national average. This was phenomenal, considering that citizens of Roseto ate all the wrong foods, smoked cigars, were overweight, drank red wine and worked in the toxic environment of the slate quarries. There was no suicide, alcoholism or drug addiction, no one was on welfare and there was no crime.

> Researchers found that the happiest people are those that have a tribe, and that isolation and loneliness contribute to major health risks.

They practiced a family-centered life, putting family needs first. There were strong marriage and family connections, with many generations living under the same roof. These connections extended beyond the family to the members of the community, and people cared for and looked out for each other. They believed in God. They experienced relatively low stress by placing all worries in God's hands and knew friends and family were there to help.

Over the years, as the community of Roseto moved away from living the slower, simpler life and adopted the modern ways of striving and competition, rushing and lack of connection, their risk for heart attacks increased. Their community began to resemble others across the country, reflecting the same issues as the rest of the nation. What can we learn from this? That rushing has negative impacts on our life, and a slower pace allows for greater connection, which has social, emotional and physical benefits. The Roseto community of older times seemed to enjoy life, valued family and community relationships with faith, and trusted that they would be taken care of. They lived an authentic life and did not fear the judgement of others for their lifestyle decisions.

Ask yourself: Do you have the supports and resources you need to move confidently towards the life you want to create?

Suzanne Colmer, owner and creator of Your Shop Girl Image Consulting, lives motivational speaker Jim Rohn's quote that we are an average of the five people we spend the most time with. She is surrounded by an incredible network of female entrepreneurs and her family. Her three-year-old daughter pushes her to remember to have fun, focus on what matters and be a better business person. Suzanne's clients have all had a recent change in their life, triggering them to grow and value the opportunity of focusing time and energy on themselves. These women, Suzanne and her clients are aware and asking for what they need and seeking their tribe for support.

Suzanne also disclosed that her workouts are key to keeping her centered, and recently her naturopath wrote on a prescription pad, "Two rigorous workouts and one balanced and calm." She wished that more people not only received prescriptions like this but also held themselves accountable to that practice.

Your vibe attracts your tribe. Do your tribes support you? Are they composed of people who love who you are and have your best interests at heart? Do you enjoy spending time with the people in your life? What might need to change?

1. Find Your Tribe

Surround yourself with people who have the same energetic vibration as you. Remember, you are the average of the five people you spend the most time with so be selective. Expand your awareness and set the intention to find a community group that resonates with who you are: Your goals and interests. I suggest finding a tribe online as well as through meetups. Listen to your intuition, both for good matches and to alert you to the possibility that a group is not for you.

2. Say "Yes, I'm In"

I have a friend who, when asked if he would like to participate in an activity, pauses for a moment, and after a moment of consideration, most often says "Yes, I'm in." I admire his willingness to take risks and engage in life with such enthusiasm and energy. I love the free spiritedness of children and their willingness to fully engage in what they are doing, and my friend's affirmative and positive approach to life reminds me of that childlike exuberance for life. Most days, he seemed unruffled at work, and I wondered how much his willingness to say "yes" and break out of the norm was responsible for his inner peace

Dr. David Elkind, author of the book *The Hurried Child: Growing Up Too Fast Too Soon*, says our children's spontaneous play time is being replaced by hectic schedules of extracurricular activities.

During free play, children use curiosity and imagination and these are actually antidotes to busyness.

Increasing academic pressure on children, beginning as early as kindergarten, has resulted in less time for play and the arts. According to the National Institutes of Mental Health 25% of 13 to 18 year olds are suffering from anxiety and stress. The Yale Center for Emotional Intelligence surveyed 22,000 high school students and they reported feeling stress, fatigue and boredom the majority of the time. We are raising our children to follow in our footsteps.

One positive approach to managing our children's stress is the trend toward mindfulness in education. It is an attempt to slow children down and have them pay attention to the present moment. The benefits of mindfulness are a reduction in stress and anxiety, increased self-regulation and focus, better sleep and improved academic performance.

Ask yourself:

- Am I willing to try something new? Can I say, "Yes, I'm in," next time someone asks me to stretch my comfort zone?
- What activity do you engage in or have strayed away from that fosters the element of play?

- Are you willing to find the time to participate in that activity in the near future? Take the next step.
- If you are a parent, is there an opportunity to reduce your child's extracurricular obligations and replace that time with spontaneous play or free time?

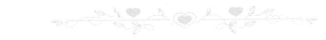

"All grownups were once children but only few of them remember it."

—ANTOINE DE SAINT-EXUPERY

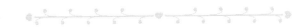

3. Ask for Help and Be a Good Receiver

Seek support from professionals who specialize in the issues you need support with. This could be within your professional organization or in your community. Ask your friends for recommendations or get a referral from your doctor. Be tenacious in finding the person who is the perfect fit of experience and personality.

Helpers are better at giving than receiving and I challenge you to practice being a good receiver. When you receive a compliment or a friend offers to buy you lunch, just say "thank you". No explanation necessary and no need to immediately set up a reciprocal arrangement to pay them back with a similar treat.

We could all learn a few things about living in the moment, unconditional love and receiving from our pets. Being a pet owner encourages you to keep your heart open and lowers your stress, cortisol levels and blood pressure. Animals don't worry about what's happening beyond the present moment. They are just happy to be. My cats and dog seem to know when is the perfect time to race around the house, for no apparent reason, providing me with entertainment and a much-needed reason to laugh. I invite you to be open to loving unconditionally, living in the moment and being open to receiving love and support.

4. Find a Mentor

A mentor is someone you admire, often doing what you would like to be doing and can provide support and advice to move you forward, especially at times when you are feeling doubt or are unsure in which direction to proceed. Is there someone in your organization you look up to or who is doing the job you would like to do? Do you need a mentor in another aspect of your life, not related to your career? Assess your needs and set the intention to find the perfect mentor.

5. Who Has Your Back?

Wendy Lantz is a social worker working with adults that have a wide variety of medical diagnoses. She provides a spectrum of care from assisting families with housing needs and connecting them to community resources to helping individuals adjust to new medical diagnoses and end-of-life planning. What I learned from Wendy was that she is able to slow down and spend time with her clients, giving her clients what they need. She became a social worker later in life and through experience she has become skilled at striking the balance between her personal and professional life. Wendy credits her success to having a supportive husband, autonomy and flexibility in her schedule and taking the time to self-reflect and journal. She says everybody needs a cheerleader and the question is not "How do you do it?" but rather "How can I help?"

It's not just our clients and family members that need a cheerleader. We also need a cheerleader for support and help in our job and in our lives and particularly if we are committed to making a change. An accountability partner or partners can help you stay the course and honour your commitment to change. When we decide to make a change, our ego turns up the negative self-talk, making us doubt our ability to meet our goal.

Find a person who is interested in being your accountability partner. They could be a friend, co-worker or anyone you intuitively know is a match. You will have greater success if they can relate to you and your goal. Agree to meet regularly and share specifics about your goals with a plan of scheduled tasks to be completed. You can help each other when you are lagging, and can provide each other a good dose of reality or a swift kick to keep moving.

Miranda deRoux, BSW, had some advice for new social work grads. She suggested an accountability partner to protect yourself from burnout and compassion fatigue. Miranda said we don't often know when we are over-extended and that having an arrangement with an accountability partner who knows you can help prevent the drift into doing too much. She said agree to let each other know if you see signs of overextending and that you will take the information seriously enough to follow up with some self-care. The agreement is to listen and respond. Miranda is presently taking a much-needed break from social work for her own well-being. She worked with addicts at a methadone clinic and as an addiction counsellor in the safe needle van with the AIDS Network. She decided to take a year away from social work, moved to British Columbia to hike and pursue her dream of producing a harp CD.

Whether you are a seasoned veteran or relatively new in your career being aware of how the demands of the job are affecting you sometimes requires a caring friend or co-worker to share their observations with you. It's up to you to take the next step.

Ponder this: Do you have a goal in mind that scares you just a little bit and you could benefit from an accountability partner? Would having an agreement with a co-worker or friend who would honestly let you know if they saw signs of burnout be of value to you?

Do you have an individual in mind that you could approach about being your accountability partner for the pursuit of a goal or to support you in your well-being as it relates to your job demands?

Contact the person or persons and choose a date to meet and discuss the possibility of an accountability partnership or as someone who has your best interests at heart. Who is your cheerleader?

6. Nurture Your Friendships

The earliest research of the fight-or-flight stress responses was derived from men's reactions only. When sociologists added women to the research, they found that women built relationships to manage stress. This became known as "tend and mend", and is not exclusively a female response to stress since we display aspects of both male and female characteristics. Women generally communicate with their friends, sharing their concerns as a way to cope with stress, and some men may also confide in their friends. I urge you to develop quality friendships for social and emotional well-being, outside of work. If you do choose to socialize with friends from work, limit conversation about work in your off hours to a specific time frame and focus on other interests and pursuits.

7. Lead with Your Heart

The term *cardiac coherence* describes the synchronization between the brain and the heart, and the result is optimal functioning of the body and a state of well-being. When we reach cardiac coherence, the heart secretes a hormone known as the bonding hormone oxytocin, which produces a state of peace and safety. In this peaceful state, we perceive situations more positively and naturally we feel good. By taking care of our well-being, we positively impact those around us.

Currently, there is a research being conducted that involves groups of people practicing cardiac coherence to create global change called the Global Coherence Initiative Project. Learn more about the project at www.heartmath.org. The HeartMath organization also facilitates workshops for individuals and teachers about how to reach cardiac coherence personally and then use it in their classrooms.

Practice slow breathing as that impacts your autonomic nervous system and slows you down. It also creates a feeling of being centered, grounded, induces a feeling of peace and results in cardiac coherence.

8. Have Fun

When I was busy working and raising children, life flew by. I had a lot of responsibility, and I was taking life very seriously, including my exercise routines. When my mother remarked on more than one occasion that I had lost my sense of humour, I realized that I could be responsible and still allow myself to have fun.

I was bored and frustrated with fitness classes, weight training and running. My body was reacting to the stress in my life and the perceived stress of aerobic exercise, with cortisol and stubborn belly fat. I was unhappy both with myself and my appearance. Two years ago I found Zumba, the total workout dance fitness party based on salsa and Latin dance moves choreographed to upbeat Latin and world rhythms, and I was hooked after my first class. It was fun! In the beginning, I was self-conscious and awkward, shaking both my upper and lower body because I wasn't used to moving in such a loose and flexible manner.

I believe women, me included, have lost some fluidity in their hips, symbolic of femininity, as we pursued careers and success in a more masculine manner. Unresolved emotions are stored as toxins in our body tissues and most often within our hips, the part of our body that is associated with change and moving forward in our lives according to Louise Hay in *Heal Your Body*. Dr. Christiane Northrup, author of *Making Life Easy*, believes shaking and physical movement encourages our body to let go of those emotions and toxins. Is it any wonder participants are committed to their classes, and that Zumba has become popular the world over?

At the studio I attend, Shake It Off in Guelph, there is a sense of community and belonging and it's quite apparent that the dynamic duo, Carlos Henriquez and Stephanie Dean, who operate the studio are truly living their passion. Together they have created an unforgettable partnership and while they like to have fun they are serious in their commitment to the success of the studio and genuinely care for the members and each other. I love the atmosphere. I have fun "working out" in an environment of inclusivity and support and I consider the members and instructors at this club part of my tribe.

Playlist

Affirm daily, as many times as you like: I am flourishing. I am health, wealth, joy, love and success.

1. Find your tribes online and in your community. Intend to meet new people, join a meetup and introduce yourself to someone new. Do it.
2. Read *The Code of the Extraordinary Mind* by Vishen Lakhiani and act on anything in the book that resonates with you.

3. Who is your accountability partner? Schedule some regular meeting times. Put them on your calendar.
4. Find a way to introduce more fun into your life.

Inspiration and Wisdom of Others

Books

- *This Time I Dance!: Creating the Work You Love* by Tama Kieves
- *The Code of the Extraordinary Mind* by Vishen Lakhiani
- *Zero Limits: The Secret Hawaiian System for Wealth, Health, Peace, and More* by Joe Vitale

Websites

- www.mindvalley.com—transformational education
- www.mindmovies.com—digital affirmations
- www.thesecret.tv—movie about manifesting what you want using the power of your subconscious mind
- www.theabundancefactormovie.com—movie featuring experts on the subject of abundance and prosperity
- www.heartmath.org

"Life is a series of near misses. But a lot of what we ascribe to luck is not luck at all. It's seizing the day and accepting responsibility for our future."

—HOWARD SCHULTZ

How does taking care of ourselves make a positive change in the world? Turn the page.

"You are invited by life to elect yourself a spiritual leader and to take office today. What does a spiritual leader say? A spiritual leader does not say, 'Follow me.' A spiritual leader says, 'I'll go first.' Decide to take the oath: I promise to 'go first' in demonstrating forgiveness, compassion, understanding, generosity, kindness, cheerfulness, positivity and love."

—NEALE DONALD WALSCH

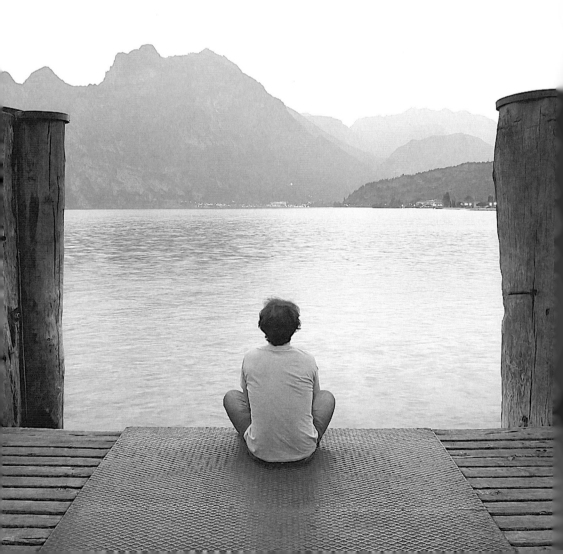

CHAPTER FIVE

STARTING WITH THE (WOMAN) MAN IN THE MIRROR

1. You First

Take the oath and assume the office of a spiritual leader today. "You first" implies you go first and others will follow, not because you ask them to, but because they are inspired by your confidence and actions. They observe how you live your life, and that you demonstrate the traits of forgiveness, compassion, understanding, generosity, cheerfulness, positivity and love and they will want what you have. Take charge of your life and commit to your goals. Be decisive, determined and seek support from your tribe, accountability partner or mentor in moving your life forward. Step into the responsibility of being a leader and lead by example.

2. Align your thoughts, words and actions

Just as we teach people how to treat us, we also show people what we value by how we speak and act. When our thoughts, words and actions are in alignment we achieve our goals with ease and speed. If our actions are not consistent with our words we lose credibility and respect from our co-workers, clients, family members and friends. What we value should be evident by our use of language and demonstrated by our behaviour. Align yourself with those who are like minded for support and inspiration. I have found that it's beneficial to keep my thoughts to myself unless I am confident I am speaking to a person who is supportive of me and my belief system.

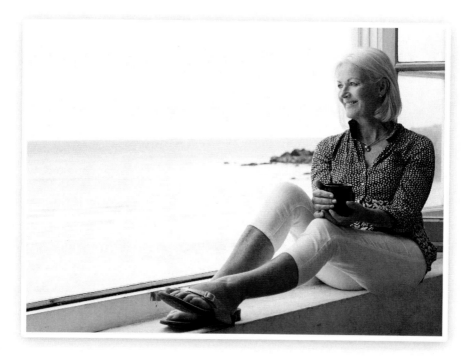

An individual I interviewed, who believes in her own well-being and that of her employees while providing a place of silence, relaxation and wellness, is Mylisa Henderson. Mylisa is the Director of Marketing and Sales at the Scandinave Spa, Blue Mountain and she's in partnership with the community and believes in being an ambassador of the region. She believes a positive outlook and concern for the well-being of other people creates a community of positivity and intends the spa to provide an escape among trees, water and vistas. Her philosophy of well-being is evident with her staff as they are offered opportunities for massages and passes for friends and spouses. The staff participates in health and wellness activities during the off season to rebuild energy and also visit local community venues so they are able to speak with authority to clientele about the Collingwood Area. Mylisa's words and actions are in alignment with her belief in wellness and she and the Scandinave Spa are leaders in encouraging personal and community wellness.

3. Learn to Play

Take a well-deserved break from the seriousness and busyness of life and let go. Engaging in activities where we can just be ourselves and act spontaneously brings us joy. Our body is flooded with endorphins and we let the responsibilities of the day melt away. When we are engaged and having fun, we feel good. Our involvement in activities that are joyful encourages others to join in, pursue endeavours that bring them joy and raises our personal and collective energetic vibration.

4. Be You

Who among us isn't doing the best we're capable of, with the understanding we have? It's freeing to just be who you are and have the freedom to choose what you want to do, where you go and with whom, regardless of other people's opinion. Allow yourself to live without the self-judgment and criticism and accept who you are, flaws and all. You are perfect just as you are, unique in your personality, skills and experience and doing the best with what you have. There is freedom in relaxing and just being you!

5. Where are You Going?

- Sharpen you focus and keep your eyes on the prize. Do you know where you are headed?
- Revisit your goals and your ideal life scenario. What do you need to adjust?
- Do you have time in your day to focus on what you want and need?
- What inspired action do you need to take today, each day, to improve your life?
- Are you balanced in your body, feeling calm and centered?
- Are you focused on all aspects of your well-being?
- Look back over the playlists for the previous chapters, and review and revise if necessary. Life is a process, always evolving and so our plans also shift. Don't get stuck on what you think should happen, be open to possibilities.

6. Make Conscious Choices

Give some thought to why you make the choices you do. Are they a habit or do you make choices consciously?

I challenge you to make your choices based on what you value and what you believe so that your thoughts, words and actions are in alignment.

Making conscious choices is being authentic and focused, and through your commitment and confidence, you will encourage others to do the same.

7. Get Gritty

The term *grit* refers to the passion and perseverance an individual has to achieve a long-term goal, regardless of challenges and obstacles. Individuals with gritty personalities don't let a challenge get in the way of their success. When I think of grit, I think of a grain of sand and how it irritates despite it's size. The irritation is an opportunity to shift your perspective, to be relentlessly solution-focused, practice inverse paranoia and expect the best. Grit your teeth and move forward with tenacity, knowing the universe has your back. If you find yourself repeating a statement based on an unwelcome thought pattern, I find saying "up until now" following the phrase helpful. It is a way of acknowledging the release of that old conditioning.

8. Invest in People

Listen attentively and engage with the people around you. Invest in them by showing interest in what interests them. We have two ears and one mouth indicating listening over talking. People feel validated when they express their thoughts, feelings and ideas and when you focus on them by listening attentively. Mirror back to them all the good you see in them, especially when they can't see it themselves. And lastly, use the four Cs to build your relationships—cooperation, commitment and communication leading to lasting connection.

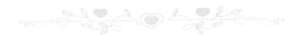

"Nobody cares how much you know until they know how much you care."

—THEODORE ROOSEVELT

Playlist

Affirm daily, as often as possible: I am flourishing. I am health, wealth, love, joy and success.

1. Create a bucket list and initiate a plan to complete some of the items on the list.
2. Write your own vision or mission statement that will help you make conscious choices providing rationale for all your decisions. State what you want to do, in the present tense, and how you will feel when you achieve that goal. There are many resources online to assist you in developing your statement.
3. Create your own affirmation related to a goal or goals. It should be personal, in the present tense and positive. Write them on a cue card and carry it with you.

Inspiration and Wisdom of Others

Books

- *Unleash the Power Within* by Tony Robbins
- *In the Meantime: Finding Yourself and the Love You Want* by Iyanla Vanzant
- *Emergence: Seven Steps for Radical Life Change* by Derek Rydall
- *The Leader Who Had No Title: A Modern Fable on Real Success in Business and Life* by Robin Sharma

Websites

- www.tonyrobbins.com
- www.myparent.com—helping parents cope with the speed of life
- www.liveyourlegend.com—local chapters to support you achieving your dreams

*What inspires you
to be the best you can be?
Turn the page.*

"Have you noticed that you feel better around some people than others? You smile more in their presence and afterward feel a little lighter, a bit more cheerful? I think of those people as 'purveyors of hope'. They help me to know that beyond every mountain I face there is a path, even if I can't see it from the valley."
—STEVE GOODIER

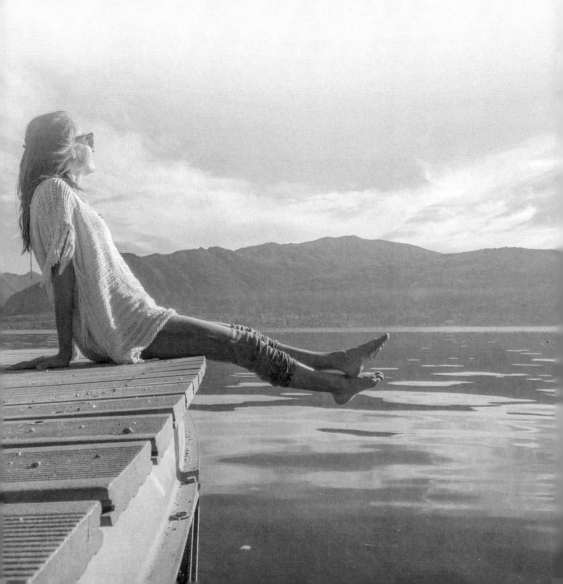

CHAPTER SIX

DON'T DIE WITH YOUR MUSIC STILL INSIDE YOU

Your greater purpose is to "be love". You also have a unique personal purpose by virtue of the fact you are here, at this time. As each thread is integral to the strength and beauty of a beautiful tapestry, so is your life and what you are here to do as only you can do.

This chapter is about being still, and silencing the chatter in your head so you can hear the guidance of your heart and spirit. This chapter is also about how your words and actions, your energy and presence inspire others. I encourage you to note where you find inspiration. By cultivating your relationship with your spirit and inner wisdom, you strengthen your connection to a higher power and open the lines of communication to receive the messages. Our body's wisdom affirms or denies the path with symptoms that, if ignored, increase in intensity.

1. Believe in Easy

Life is a gift. The present is the only time we can make choices and act as the past is behind us and the future has not yet happened. Worry is a form of prayer, so with an attitude of appreciation and anticipation, believe that life is easy. Believe in a life of ease and see everything going the way you would like. For example, see the people you interact with as accepting and supportive of your ideas and willing to help you achieve your goals and desires. Visualize even the most difficult and argumentative individual wishing you well and offering their support and also see them achieving what they desire. I use this technique when I feel apprehensive about the outcome of a meeting or presentation. This raises my energy and focuses my attention on a positive outcome. Our minds can't differentiate between what is imagined and what has happened so reinforce the positive by visualizing on the outcome you wish.

Create meaning in your life by focusing on what you want and then commit to making it happen. Have fun, play and release the struggle.

2. Establish a Morning Ritual

I find that when I follow my morning ritual, I have a calmer and more productive day. As I awaken, I take a few moments to set the intention for a good day and focus on what I need to do that day. When I drink my coffee, I spend the solitary time reading, writing, letting my mind wander and setting myself up for a good day. I walk my dog, either with my partner or by myself enjoying nature and then I use the quiet time in my hot tub to reflect on my goals. My goals are written in detail, on cue cards that I carry with me and I make adjustments and write affirmations as needed. I set the intention to take inspired action towards my goals and I take that inspired action each day.

3. Set Your Intention

Before I fall asleep, I take a moment to reflect on my day, what I appreciated and what I might have done differently. Is there someone I need to speak to and clear up any misperceptions, or issues from the day. Lastly, I take a few moments to consider "3-2-1": 3 things I am most grateful for; 2 intentions or affirmations related to my goals, either daily or long term, and 1 inspired action step I am committing to doing the next day.

4. Be Still and Listen

Meditation is the time spent in silence which enables us to listen to the guidance from our higher self. Meditation benefits us and its effect also impacts others. The Maharishi Effect, defined as 1% of the population practicing a Transcendental Meditation program in any city, reduces the crime and accident rates, and establishes a new formula for the creation of an ideal society, free from crime and problems. There have been a number of experiments conducted to prove the validity of this effect, and I refer you to Gregg Braden's book *The Spontaneous Healing of Belief* where he expands on the research.

"If we can learn to become our prayers and hopes, expressing them in our daily interactions, then together, we can create a more peaceful and loving world."

—LENEDRA J. CARROLL

5. Ask and It Will Be Given

If meditation is what we hear, then prayer is asking for what we want. There are many methods of prayer, and I urge you to find prayer that works for you. Affirmative prayer is stating what you want, present tense, as if it is already here and therefore affirming it's manifestation. I urge you to visit Unity's website for examples of affirmative prayer. I have included two prayers that I use. I also write my own affirmative prayers to assist in manifesting what I want and need.

The Serenity Prayer: God grant me the serenity to accept the things I cannot change, the courage to change the things I can and the wisdom to know the difference.

Adaptation: God grant me the serenity to accept the people I cannot change. The courage to change the one I can. And the wisdom to know it's ME. Practice the pause: Pause before judging, pause before assuming, pause before accusing and pause whenever you are about to react harshly, and you will avoid doing and saying things you will later regret.

Prayer of Loving Kindness—Metta prayer:

May all beings be peaceful.
May all beings be happy.
May all beings be safe.
May all beings awaken to the light of their true nature.
May all beings be free.

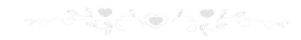

"You must ask for what you really want. Don't go back to sleep."

—RUMI

6. Notice What and Who Inspires You

Who inspires you to action? Who is doing exactly what you would like to be doing? Read a biography of an inspiring person. Sign up for daily emails from someone who inspires you and make reading it part of your daily routine. I find time to read either in the morning or before bed, and any book by Wayne Dyer is my preference. Find time to be in places that inspire you and brings you more closely to what you consider is Divine.

> Make someone's day with an act of kindness and compassion. What can you do to positively affect a person's day?

7. Make Someone's Day

Make someone's day with an act of kindness and compassion. What can you do to positively affect a person's day? Inspire someone through your action. Mother Theresa challenged us to find someone who is alone and convince them of their worth by extending love and compassion so they no longer feel alone.

"Let us always meet each other with smile, for the smile is the beginning of love."

—MOTHER THERESA

Practice random acts of kindness or pay it forward. For example, pay for the person in the car behind you when you go through the drive-through.

Create a Superstar campaign or a campaign that resonates more easily in your workplace or community. I initiated the Superstar campaign at a school to encourage students and teachers to notice people doing things that made someone smile or helped in some way. It raised the morale, as people were happy to catch others doing nice things. As teachers, we made a concentrated effort to be inclusive in our observations so everyone felt the sense of community. Would something like this work in your class, school or organization?

8. Act with Passion and Purpose

This means act with discernment and take decisive action with enthusiasm. Be open to the possibility of opportunities and set yourself up for success. Your personal purpose will make itself known to you if you listen and follow the guidance of your heart and spirit. If you are distracted and busy in life, your spirit's whisperings can't be heard so be mindful and patient.

Playlist

Affirm daily, as many times as you can: I am flourishing. I am health, wealth, love, joy and success.

1. Establish your morning ritual. Just do it.
2. Before getting out of bed in the morning, visualize a goal for 17 seconds. If you really want to ramp it up, spend 68 seconds on the goal and how you will feel when you achieve the goal. This exercise is credited to Esther and Gerry Hicks in the book *Getting into the Vortex*.
3. Practice asking and receiving using prayer and meditation.

Inspiration and Wisdom of Others

Books

- *Ask and It Is Given* by Abraham—Hicks
- *The Language of Letting Go* by Melody Beattie—daily inspirational readings
- *A Daily Dose of Sanity* by Alan Cohen—daily inspirational readings
- *Dying to Be Me: My Journey from Cancer, to Near Death, to True Healing* by Anita Moorjani
- *What If This Is Heaven?: How Cultural Myths Prevent Us from Experiencing Heaven on Earth* by Anita Moorjani
- *Left to Tell: Discovering God Amidst the Rwandan Holocaust* by Immaculée Ilibagiza
- *Inspiration: Your Ultimate Calling* by Wayne Dyer

Websites

- www.truenorthinsight.org—meditation retreats
- www.riversoundretreat.com—retreats and yoga
- www.zen12.com—online meditation for 12 minutes
- www.nealedonaldwalsch.com—daily online inspiration

"NOTHING is more expensive in your life than a closed mind and a missed opportunity."

—GERRY ROBERT

How do we put all this together?

Take a deep breath

and turn the page.

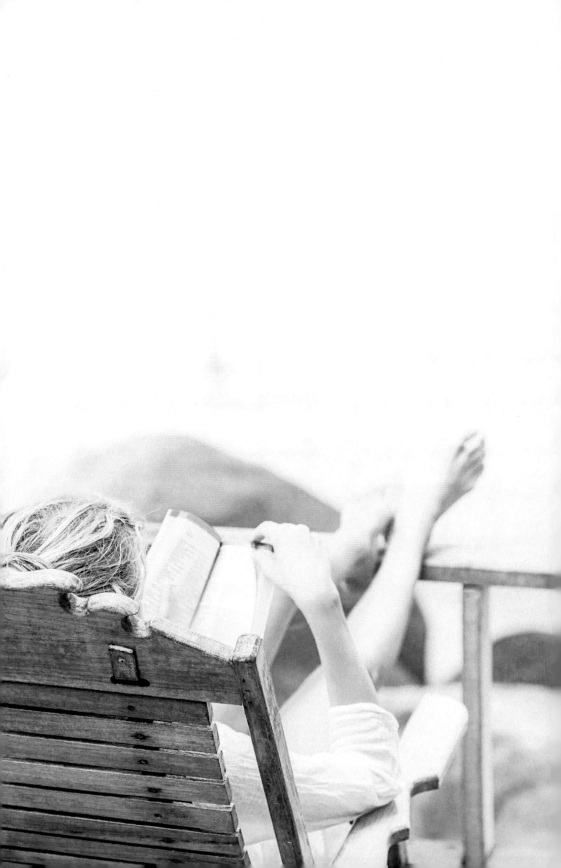

CHAPTER SEVEN

ALL IS WELL

*A*ristotle believed we all seek to flourish and that means living the good life. It is about well-being as a holistic concept—physically, emotionally, socially and spiritually, and it has to do with your own personal definition. It is a feeling and so has nothing to do with the external. **You** know if you are flourishing because you have decided what flourishing means to you. These last two chapters are about putting it all together and being in harmony with your spirit, the Earth and others.

"I believe life is a journey, often difficult and sometimes incredibly cruel, but we are well equipped for it if only we tap into our talents and gifts and allow them to blossom."

—LES BROWN

This chapter is about synergy and creating the masterpiece of your life. The sum of the whole is stronger than the individual parts. You as an individual and you are a member of a community: Family, workplace and the neighbourhood in which you live in addition to the greater communities of your city, province and country. When our body, mind and spirit is in alignment or synergy, we are healthier. We are also stronger together when we take care of our well-being, accept the help from others and encourage others to do the same.

1. Adopt an Attitude of Wabi-Sabi

The Japanese term *wabi-sabi* is essentially the appreciation for the imperfections in yourself and others. It's about accepting who we are—imperfect, unfinished and mortal—and through the passage of time, accepting and appreciating where we've been damaged and the beauty and value of those experiences. To bring wabi-sabi into our lives, we need to slow down, shift from doing to being and appreciate who we are—cracked and imperfect, however, beautiful, without feeling a need to fix and be perfect. The Japanese believe that when something has been damaged, it takes on richer character and becomes more valuable. See the beauty in the imperfection in both yourself and others.

"The more I stop trying to force outcome and simply be in the flow, the more magic that my life is meant to be, appeared. I made a decision to 'let go' and enjoy while appreciating what I was going through and where it was taking me. That is when I realized that I could control everything that I was experiencing. I simply experienced it without labeling it as bad or good, beneficial or loss, releasing all judgment and having faith."

—DIVYA VINAI SHAH

2. Practice Wabi-Sabi in the Workplace

Express your appreciation for those around you and encourage them to be the best they can be. The idea of wabi-sabi seems to contradict the philosophy of striving for perfection in the workplace. When we are valued for who we are and can be more authentic we feel more secure and that eliminates the competitiveness and power struggles. Our words and actions are in alignment with our values and that reflects our best self.

My pets' vet, Dr. Scott Gardiner, told me he rarely receives a thank-you note or a good news call from the pet owners he takes care of (that statement is accurate in that he looks after two patients, both the owner and the animal). He was not the first interviewee to highlight the fact that there is little appreciation for the jobs they do. He is able to build rapport easily with the owners and they often disclose very personal information and wonder afterwards why they shared with him. During our interview he told me that there are less limits to the care we provide humans while the extent to which he can care for an animal often has a financial limitation. I had not thought of that before. I appreciate the care and dedication he demonstrates toward me and my animals and since the interview I have made it a practice to express my appreciation to people either verbally or with thank you cards. We don't know what impacts the decisions people make each day and this was good reminder for me, after becoming aware of the parameters within which Scott has to work.

"There is a crack in everything. That's how the light gets in."

—LEONARD COHEN

3. Immerse Yourself

Be present in your body, and let life live through you. Living with the wabi-sabi approach means accepting how your life is unfolding without forcing outcomes. Be mindful and present as you focus on your actions and feelings when you are doing what you are doing. Don't rush ahead in your mind to what you must do next and that includes formulating an answer or response to someone while they are sharing with you. Enjoy the experience and immerse yourself in the activity and be respectful to others by actively listening.

4. Believe In Serendipity

When we slow down, feel good and stay in the moment, we are more open to pleasant surprises or serendipity. Believing in the occurrence of events by chance, leading to our highest good, means living with the expectation of life unfolding in beneficial ways leading to our happiness. Can you let go of specific outcomes and be open to the possibility of the universe providing opportunities that benefit and even thrill you? Notice the surprises that show up and be grateful.

"Flow can only truly be achieved when we are willing to let go of the outcome and just play."

—SANDRA TAYLOR HEDGES

5. Love and Appreciation

The more we are grateful, the more there is to be grateful about. When we make the choice to feel good and believe good things are happening, the more we notice. When we appreciate the good, more shows up to feel good about. The simplest prayer to say each day is "thank you, thank you, thank you," regardless of what's happening. Saying "thank you" no matter what is remembering that there's a reason for everything. There is a silver lining beneath the struggle even if at the time it seems impossible to conceive.

6. Lighten Up

Find your lightness of being. When I was working I tried not to take myself, my job or the circumstances of my life so seriously, and to laugh at myself when I made a mistake, as all human beings do. I also needed to recognize that while I was surrounded by the sadness of my student's situations and my own stressful personal life, I could still find the time and place to laugh. During some of my interviews, individuals shared that they employed a sort of black humour as a survival tactic. Move from a serious demeanour to a lighter, faster energy by seeking out opportunities to laugh. Watch a comedy or comedian, watch young children play, or animals frolic. Turn off the TV, especially the news and that also includes screen time and social media.

7. Go with the Flow, Be in the Flow

When we are in the flow, we are completely involved in what we are doing and time flies. Our whole being is involved and we are completely engaged using our skills to the best of our ability. Every action flows from one to the next, as do our thoughts, and our ego falls away. Going with the flow is surrendering and trusting that you will get where it is you need to get to. Aim to be in the flow and go with the flow, enjoying what you are doing at the present moment and trusting that the next moment will flow, followed by the next one, and all is well. Relinquish control and go with the flow.

"You are learning too much, remembering too much, trying too hard... relax a little bit, give life a chance to flow its own way, unassisted by your mind and effort."

—MOOJI

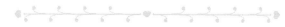

8. The Big Reveal—Develop Your Plan

During the interviews, I asked my interviewees what their definition of flourishing was and everyone provided a different answer. There were some similarities; however, there were some subtle nuances that made the answer unique to them. The definition of flourishing is personal and only you know if you are flourishing or not. This book has focused your attention on your life, through exploring your experiences and uncovering what you want and need. The underlying premise of the book is that when we focus on our own lives, we can flourish, having the time and energy to put attention on pursuing what we want. Each chapter of the book emphasized a necessary element in creating a flourishing life and they are: **F**ocus, **L**ove, **O**wnership, **U**nity, **R**esponsibility, **I**nspiration, **S**ynergy and **H**armony—**FLOURISH**.

This process can be applied specifically to resolving an issue in your life or achieving a goal. Just as easily, you can use this process to improve your life generally, and it can be used in your family, community or organization with some adaptation of the questions to fit a group's needs. Our life is so much bigger, better and grander when we put it all together, integrating all our skills, experience and learning. We also have stronger, more efficient organizations when we work cooperatively rather than competitively.

The Flourishing Process

Focus: What do I (we) want?

Clarifying questions: What do I (we) want to accomplish? Or what is my (our) goal? What is the problem I (we) would like to resolve?

Love: What do I (we) do well?

Clarifying questions: What unique skills, experience or strengths do I (we) need to focus on? What do I love that I (we) do? Is there a similar experience in my (our) past that I (we) could rely on to help me (us)?

Ownership: What's in the way?

Clarifying questions: What is the obstacle and what do I (we) need to solve the issue? What resources or information do I (we) need to make improvements in the existing condition to move forward? What behaviours have contributed to the present situation and which are mine (ours) to own and repair?

Unity: Who and what supports me (us)?

Clarifying questions: What supports or which people do I (we) need? What practices might I (we) need to put in place to encourage cooperation and an atmosphere of trust and willingness?

Responsibility: What's my (our) role and what are the steps?

Clarifying questions: What are the steps I (we) might need to consider? What is mine (ours) to do? How can I (we) be a leader? What resources or information do I (we) need to make improvements in the existing condition to move forward?

Inspiration: Why am I (are we) doing this?

Clarifying questions: Who and what might I (we) need to keep moving forward, especially if I (we) meet an obstacle? What or who will keep me (us) motivated and inspired?

Synergy: What does the plan look like?

Clarifying questions: What is the sequence of events and steps towards the goal or resolution? What is the timeline? Who does what as I (we) play to each other's strengths?

Harmony: How does this benefit others?

Clarifying questions: Are there some partners who would be willing to cooperate with me (us) to meet my (our) goal or reach a resolution? Are there organizations or community partners who would benefit from me (us) reaching my (our) goal or resolving the issue? How can I (we) contribute to the bigger vision?

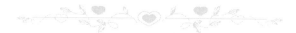

"Live with intention. Walk to the edge. Listen hard. Practice Wellness. Play with abandon. Laugh. Choose with no regret. Appreciate your friends. Continue to learn. Do what you love. Live as if this is all there is."

—MARY ANNE RADMACHER

Playlist

Affirm every day, as often as possible: I am flourishing. I am health, wealth, love, joy and success.

1. Apply the FLOURISH process and develop your plan to reach a goal or create the life of your dreams. Review your journal and tips and strategies throughout the book in addition to the resources for support. Partner with a friend and collaborate for more support.
2. Check out www.lifebookultimate.com as another option to assist in creating your best life. Jon Butcher has manifested success, happiness and fulfillment in all 12 categories of his life and turned his life into a masterpiece. You can also find an interview with him about the lifebook on Mindvalley.

Inspiration and Wisdom of Others

Books

- *It's a Meaningful Life: It Just Takes Practice* by Bo Lozoff
- *Buddha's Brain: The Practical Neuroscience of Happiness, Love, and Wisdom* by Rick Hanson

Websites

- www.optimallivingprogram.com—Brian Johnson of Philosopher's Notes and Optimize +1
- www.shoutyourjoy.com—how to life joyfully

"This is a marathon in life. You can't be sprinting all the time or else you wear yourself out. You have to make sure you're taking care of yourself, keeping yourself grounded and not letting every little thing get you worked up."

—BRIAN MOYNIHAN

Now that we have it together, how do we keep it together with everyone else? Turn the page.

"*The opportunity of our times is for each one of us to understand at a very personal level, that we can have a profound impact on the world in which we live. The greatest possibilities for global transformation exist in the fabric of our individual lives.*"

—LENEDRA J. CARROLL

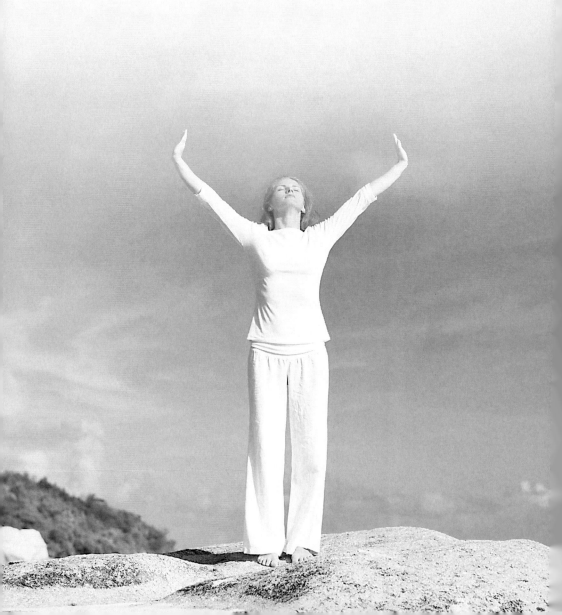

CHAPTER EIGHT

THE CHOICE IS YOURS

The word harmony conjures up thoughts about music and the coordinated effect of all instruments playing together. To make beautiful music, everyone plays their best and pays attention to the arrangement for their instrument. To live harmoniously means to live in cooperation with everything and everyone that surrounds us, while each of us uses our unique skills and plays our part.

Harmony has to be within each of us first as we move authentically in our lives, doing what we believe we are here to do and we are content, if not happy. We mean what we say and act consistently with what we believe and that contributes to creating harmony within our relationships in our homes, workplace and communities. We are spiritual beings having a human experience, and are in alignment with our spirit, recognizing our oneness and the connection to each other and to God (Universe, Spirit, the Divine, Higher Power etc). This chapter is simply about being.

Eight Ways to Be

1. Be Patient

From *A Course in Miracles* comes the expression, "with infinite patience comes immediate results". *A Course in Miracles* was scribed by Helen Schucman and is a metaphysical self-study book. Be open to possibility and in the meantime, choose to live life easy while you are waiting to discover your purpose. You will be guided to it by listening to your heart and body while fully engaging in life while you wait.

I love the book *The Four Agreements* by Don Miguel Ruiz to be used as a guide for life. The four simple statements are easy to remember, however, not always so easy to implement. They are: Be impeccable with your word, don't take anything personally, don't make assumptions and always do your best. These statements suit any circumstance, and when you apply them, the outcome is more harmonious than conflicted.

"We recognize our own mortality and we are reminded that in the fleeting time we have on this Earth, what matters is not wealth, or status, or power or fame, but, rather, how we have loved, and what small part we have played in making the lives of other people better."

—BARACK OBAMA

2. Be Love

This also is simple and not always easy. Expand your heart and demonstrate love in all that you do and remember everything is love or a cry for love. Choose love not fear. By shining the light on what scares you, it loses its power.

3. Be Happy

Emily Fletcher, founder of zivaMIND, the first online meditation training, spoke at Mindvalley's A-Fest and made reference to the "I'll Be Happy When" syndrome. She said happiness is a choice and we can choose to be happy now regardless of what's happening. If you fall into the "I'll Be Happy When" Syndrome, you'll always be striving for a certain circumstance in the future and therefore not happy where you are presently. Your focus is on what's lacking instead of appreciating what is.

Would you rather be right or would you rather be happy? This question invites us to be in the moment and appreciate the people we are in a relationship with. We could judge and correct them or remain silent and decide making the comment is not worth our mutual happiness. We can opt to mirror back to them goodness and peace and show them love instead of what might be lacking.

"Happiness is not a destination. It is a method of life."

—BURTON HILLS

4. Be Generous

Give your time and energy from a place of fulfillment and eagerness to help, and not from a place of lack. When we take care of ourselves first, we have lots of energy and interest in helping and supporting others. The law of circulation, or reap what you sow, means what we give, we receive. When we give from a place of lack, struggle, fatigue and out of obligation, receiving what we want is challenging. When we give from fullness and love, we have infinite time and energy and receiving is easy. Consider tithing, the practice of giving 10% as a spiritual tithe and enforcing the law of circulation financially.

5. Be Joy

Joy is a feeling of happiness and pleasure. The word *happiness* comes from the Greek concept of *eudaimonia,* which refers to the good life or flourishing. Make joy your goal as it consists of both happiness and pleasure. Look for opportunities to be joyful and to rejoice, therefore raising your vibration to the highest frequency as identified on the emotional scale by Abraham Hicks. You encourage others to raise their vibration simply by being near you.

6. Be Peace

As interdependent beings, when we are being peace we create a ripple effect and that calmness and quiet positively impacts those around us. Be peace in the eye of the storm. Inner peace comes with acceptance of what is. Although there are changes we might like to see in our personal and professional lives, we need to make peace with what is and then look to make improvements from a place of positivity or the very least neutrality. By tweaking our focus slightly, we move from being problem-focused and complaining to solution-focused. We work with the circumstances of our lives as they unfold so as not to cause our thoughts, words and actions to become chaotic.

7. Be Enthusiastic

Enthusiasm means "God within", so being enthusiastic means we are joyful and energized through our connection to something greater than ourselves. When we are passionate about life, our energetic vibration attracts more circumstances to be passionate about. Believing in something greater than ourselves reduces our fears and anxiety, we have faith we are not alone and are supported on our spiritual path. Be enthusiastic and embrace who you are and where you are and that way of being will be infectious.

8. Be One

Do no harm to others with either your words or actions. Do as the quote suggests and treat others as the spiritual divine creatures they are. One of the interpretations of the word " Namaste" means "the Divine in me bows to the Divine in you". Namaste is used as a greeting that shows respect and a recognition of our equality. As sparks of the Divine we are inherently good and deserve to live a life that is flourishing.

"*Beginning today, treat everyone you meet as if they were going to be dead by midnight. Extend to them all the care, kindness and understanding you can muster, and do it with no thought of any reward. Your life will never be the same again.*"

—OG MANDINO

Affirm I am okay right here, right now and release the worry and fear that you are not. By raising your vibration, you encourage others to raise theirs and encourage coherence between the hearts.

Playlist

Affirm every day, as often as possible: I am flourishing. I am health, wealth, love, joy and success.

1. Be happy now. Set the intention daily. Happiness is a state of mind that you choose.
2. Be of service. Each morning, ask how you may serve. *A Course in Miracles* offers this suggestion to be asked each morning. Where would You have me go? What would You have me do? What would You have me say, and to whom?
3. Be involved in your local and global community. Take responsibility and be a leader.
4. What do you need to do to feel you are leading a flourishing life?

Inspiration and Wisdom of Others

Books

- *Making Life Easy: A Simple Guide to a Divinely Inspired Life* by Christiane Northrup
- *10% Happier* by Dan Harris
- *The Architecture of All Abundance* by Lenedra J. Carroll
- *The Greatness Guide* and *The Greatness Guide Book 2* by Robin Sharma

Websites

- www.agapelive.com—Michael Beckwith's international spiritual centre
- www.lifehack.org—tips for health and happiness
- www.zivameditation.com

"If everyone is moving forward together, then success takes care of itself."
—HENRY FORD

Where do we go from here?

What's next?

Turn the page.

"The opportunity of our times is for each one of us to understand at a very personal level, that we can have a profound impact on the world in which we live. The greatest possibilities for global transformation exist in the fabric of our individual lives."
—LENEDRA J. CARROLL

END NOTES: NOTHING MOVES UNTIL YOU DO

"We need to imagine a world at peace, and then work backward from there. The world can only be at peace when more of its people are fed, housed, and educated; when more of its people are given the medical care they need; when more of its women are free; when more of its opportunities are available for more of its population; and when more of its resources are shared equitably. These things wouldn't just 'be nice'—they're essential keys to a survivable future."

—MARIANNE WILLIAMSON

As the title suggests, we need to move to affect change in our world. This chapter provides hope for the future with ideas from deeply passionate professional people, so what could be more relevant and impactful? Françoise Mathieu, of the TEND Academy, says we are role modeling balance for our children and there is room for improvement. She would like to see poverty eradicated and increased literacy which is challenging because in our society, we have individuals and families who are underprivileged, under-resourced and affected by multigenerational trauma. Helpers are drained by repeat visits due to multigenerational family issues, the opiate epidemic, attachment disorder and adverse childhood trauma. We have made some improvements however, our lifestyle, work and societal issues are costing us emotionally and physically. Let's continue what we started, and remain focused on our health and our dreams. As we take care of ourselves we transform our lives, those we are in relationship with and together we help to heal the world.

The following suggestions are courtesy of my interviewees, blended with the ideas presented in this book. I am extremely grateful for their thoughtfulness and willingness to share so openly in the hopes of making a difference for all of us in our professions, for our children and the health of the world.

Together Can We Agree to…?

- Slow down and be aware of what we need and what we want and make those a priority.
- Focus on our well-being—physical, mental, emotional, social and spiritual—so as to achieve some balance not only within our bodies but in our lives and role model well-being for our children.
- Strike a balance between our personal and profession lives and our home and individual time.
- Seek emotional support for our triggers so as not to harm or re-wound those around us, particularly those of us who work with children, as it is an honour and responsibility.
- Own our stories and end the cycle of addiction and multigenerational trauma and take responsibility for our lives.
- Commit to raising empathetic, compassionate and respectful citizens by role modeling gentleness, respect, love and forgiveness to our children and seek parenting support when necessary without fear of judgment.
- Teach children how to "be" in the world by teaching emotional and financial literacy, the art of communicating, self-responsibility, accountability and empower them to feel and express their feeling.

END NOTES: NOTHING MOVES UNTIL YOU DO

In Our Schools, Can We...?

- Focus on supporting students in building grit and emotional regulation and support authentic communication in an emotionally and physically safe environment.
- Empower our students by building self-worth and encouraging love of self and others so as to develop compassion and confidence leading to life success and reduce incidents of violence based on intolerance.
- Renew the focus on arts, culture and physical activity to teach empathy through music, storytelling and play, highlighting curiosity and imagination.
- Educate our children about holistic well-being (mental, physical, spiritual, emotional and social) and how to manage a life in balance therefore reducing the risk of burnout, compassion fatigue, PTSD and substance and alcohol abuse in the future.
- Explain honestly about drug and alcohol use, addiction and the impact on the body and personal relationships.
- Train and support teachers and administrators about trauma leading to trauma-sensitive schools and advocate for the use of the ACE study to better support our students.
- Encourage the art of face-to-face communication rather than connection through social media and reduce the detrimental effects of isolation, loneliness, comparison and low self-worth.

In Our Post-Secondary, Continuing Education and Professional Development Programs, Can We...?

- Allow more opportunity for coop and job shadowing and have honest conversations about the reality of the "helping" jobs and demands and provide more specific training to promote better job readiness.

- Emphasize the importance of personal well-being, particularly as it relates to the risk of burnout, compassion fatigue and vicarious trauma.
- Educate about the effects of mental health disorders, addiction and drug use on individuals, relationships and society.
- In relevant professions, provide opportunities for de-briefing after emotional incidents and encourage and support counselling with trained professionals.
- Encourage and provide mandatory debriefing and ongoing scheduled check-ins for emotional health in professions where there is risk of emotional injury.
- Provide appropriate and effective support to address needs in Employee Assistance Programs.
- Focus on supporting professionals with appropriate training related to trauma, addiction , mental health issues, compassion fatigue, PTSD, burnout, grief and loss as it relates to the responsibilities of their job and supporting the helpers.

Given our societal concerns with addiction and the opiate crisis, poverty and literacy, perhaps as empathetic citizens we should all focus on these concerns and what we can do individually and collectively. It is our responsibility to take care of our health first, and support each other in being as well as possible so we role model healthy behaviour for our children and lead by example. Together we can do this and change the paradigm that has us sacrificing our own lives for others leading to more burnout and overloading the systems that employ us. When we are healthier and happier we have more energy and time to help others and together we can make a difference in the world. Let's make the shift and commit to doing it differently for all our sakes. Commit to say, "Yes, I'm in," and as Carlos from Shake It Off says, "Let's do this!"

"Here's to the crazy ones. The misfits. The rebels. The troublemakers. The round pegs in the square holes. The ones who see things differently. They're not fond of rules. And they have no respect for the status quo. You can quote them, disagree with them, glorify or vilify them. About the only thing that you can't do is ignore them. Because they change things. They push the human race forward. And while some may see them as the crazy ones, we see genius. Because the people who are crazy enough to think they can change the world, are the ones who do."

—APPLE'S "THINK DIFFERENT" AD

ACKNOWLEDGEMENTS

Thank you to Gerry Robert and the team at Black Card Books. Without their support and expertise this book would never have been published. A special thank you and acknowledgment to Marybeth Haines for her guidance and support in all facets of the book publishing process. Although I haven't listed all of you at BCB who gave of your time and energy to this book, know I am extremely grateful to each one of you.

To Tom: Thank you for the love, encouragement and support you have demonstrated over the last year for without it, this book would not have been possible. I am so very grateful for your willingness and generosity in providing financial support and the time and freedom to write. I am so thankful you are in my life and on this path with me.

I am so grateful to my family: My children, mother, brother, sister and brother-in-law, and to my dad's presence from another realm. Your love, support and encouragement has been very much appreciated.

To those wise authors, and particularly the works of Wayne Dyer, who have inspired and guided me with their words all my life and during the writing process from beginning to end.

Thank you to my tribe, those cheerleaders of support: Julie, Becky, Merrilynn, Linda, Mitch, Bruce, Louise, and De. There are many others who expressed interest and motivated me during the times I needed it most.

Thank you to Amber Richmond for the patience you took with me to create such beautiful photographs.

Thank you very much to my sponsors who chose to partner with me and the book. Your financial and personal support is very much appreciated: Bay Gardens Funeral Homes, Kilbride and Associates, Paul Gazzola Mortgage Associates and Dr Scott Gardiner of Guelph Lakes and Woodlawn Vet practices.

ACKNOWLEDGEMENTS

And finally, to my interviewees:

- Lynne Atkinson—Funeral Director, Bay Gardens Funeral Home, Hamilton
- Becky Beausaert, PhD—Sessional Instructor, Brock, Laurier, Guelph Universities
- Luke Boudreau—Director of Chancellors Way Medical Arts Centre, Guelph
- Sandy Brooks—MSW Regional Implementation Coordinator at CAMH, Hamilton
- Susan Bushell—AAMET EFT Trainer/Level Three Practitioner, Guelph
- Suzanne Colmer—Owner, Your Shop Girl, Toronto
- Tom Dagg—Retired Secondary School Principal, Upper Grand District School Board
- Stephanie Dean—Zumba Instructor, Shake It Off Studio, Guelph
- Miranda deRoux—BSW, Abbotsford, BC
- Merrilynn Downey—Kilbride and Associates, Palmerston
- Brad Enright—Captain, Firefighter, Woodstock
- Andrea Farrell—Paramedic, Toronto Paramedic Service, Toronto
- Dr. Scott Gardiner—Vet/Owner of Woodlawn Veterinary Hospital and Guelph Lake Veterinary Hospital, Guelph
- Paul Gazzola—Guelph Mortgage Associates, Guelph
- Marino Gazzola—Retired Police Sergeant, Guelph Police Department, Guelph
- Leanne Giavedoni—Physiotherapist, doTERRA Essential Oils, Hamilton
- Mylisa Henderson—Director of Marketing and Sales, Scandinave Spa Blue Mountain

- Carlos Henriquez—Zumba Instructor, Owner, Shake It Off Studio, Guelph
- Andi Jakowlew—Osteopath, Guelph
- Eileen Kilbride—Kilbride and Associates, Palmerston
- Wendy Lantz—MSW, Community Social Worker, Woodstock
- Amy McCartney—Funeral Director, Manager, Bay Gardens Funeral Home, Hamilton
- Erin McInnis—Community Service Coordinator, Hospice Wellington, Guelph
- Madeleine Marentette—Owner, Grail Springs Retreat and Spa, Bancroft
- Françoise Mathieu—TEND Academy, Kingston
- Elizabeth Mitchell—Elementary Teacher, Halton District School Board
- Dr. Amber Moore—ND, Townsend Naturopathic Clinic, Burlington
- Mitch Nadon—Media Intelligence, Animal Rescue, C4P, Aurora
- Kelly Romanick—Moksha Yoga Studio Owner, Massage Therapist and Osteopath Student, Guelph
- Angela Spiller—RN, ONA Bargaining Unit President and Local Coordinator, Hamilton
- Terra Teas—Hamilton
- Julie Whitely—Insurance Agent, Guelph
- Trevor Wright—Wright and Associates Financial Services, Guelph

Thank you all for your time and energy for without your input this book would not have been written. It was truly an honour to get to know you. Words cannot express how much you impacted me with what you shared so openly about your lives, careers and experiences. Each interview further renewed my faith in humankind to be in the presence of such caring human beings and devoted professionals. Namaste.

Kilbride & Associates
Practice in Children's Mental Health

*A unique private practice in Mental Health
Offered by Eileen Kilbride and Merrilynn Downey
Specializing in Attachment, Trauma and Animal-assisted Therapy*

Consultation • Assessment • Individual, Group and Family Counselling

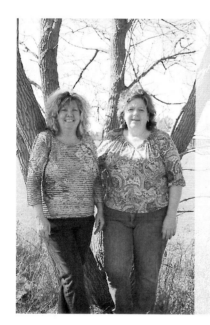

Professional Training and Consultation

We specialize in training related to Trauma Informed practice: Understanding and Supporting Youth with Severe Emotional & Behavioural Challenges and other related topics.
Our training is suitable for staff from mental health, child welfare, residential treatment centres and schools and can be customized to meet your needs.

Specialized Services Include:

Eye Movement Desensitization Reprocessing (EMDR)
Circle of Security (TM)
Cognitive Behaviour Therapy (CBT)
Dialectical Behaviour Therapy (DBT)
School Observation
Advocacy, Home Based Services
Case Conferencing, Service Coordination

*www.kilbrideandassociates.com
+519 477 1340
eileenkilbride@hotmail.com*

BAY GARDENS & BAYVIEW
funerals, cremations, cemetery & mausoleum

EVERY *life* TELLS A *story.*
CELEBRATE *yours.*

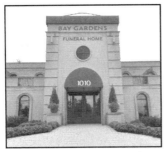

BAY GARDENS FUNERAL HOME

1010 Botanical Drive
Burlington
+905 527-0405

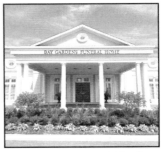

BAY GARDENS FUNERAL HOME

947 Rymal Road East
Hamilton
+905 574-0405

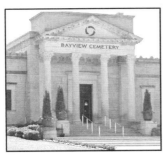

BAYVIEW CEMETERY, CREMATORY & MAUSOLEUM

740 Spring Gardens Road
Burlington
+905 522-5466

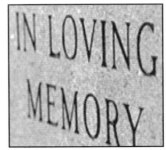

BAYVIEW MONUMENTS

1028 Botanical Drive
Burlington
+905 529-1441

www.BayGardens.ca

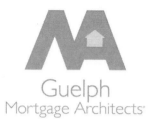

Guelph
Mortgage Architects

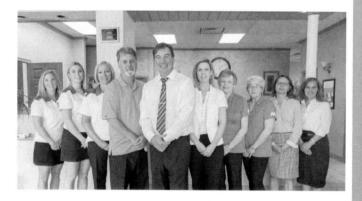

WE CAN HELP MAKE YOUR DREAM HOME, A REALITY

We believe that every customer deserves the best care and service when purchasing or refinancing the home of their dreams. We're here to serve your mortgage needs and have what it takes to make a difference in your next mortgage transaction. Our experienced team at Guelph Mortgage Architects looks forward to helping you achieve your financial and homeownership goals.

Paul Gazzola, AMP
Mortgage Broker, Lic.#M08005234
Brokerage # 12336
www.tobemortgagefree.com

Buying a home is an exciting time! You're about to take a big step so you'll definitely need some advice from a mortgage professional.

We'll give you the facts your bank won't tell you about financing your next purchase.

Apply Today
www.tobemortgagefree.com

GUELPH MORTGAGE ARCHITECTS
3 Speedvale Ave. East
Guelph, Ont.
N1H 1J2
+519 763-6436

www.tobemortgagefree.com

OTHER BOOKS RECOMMENDED BY BLACK CARD BOOKS

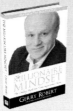

The Millionaire Mindset
How Ordinary People Can Create Extraordinary Income
Gerry Robert
ISBN: 978-1-927411-00-1

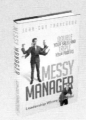

Messy Manager
Double Your Sales And Triple Your Profits
Jean-Guy Francoeur
ISBN: 978-0-9786-663-0-9

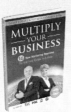

Multiply Your Business
10 New Marketing Realities for the Real Estate Industries
Gerry Robert &
Theresa Barnabei, DREC
ISBN: 978-1-77204-774-5

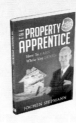

The Property Apprentice
How To EARN While You LEARN
Jochen Siepmann
ISBN (Softcover): 978-1-77204-453-9
ISBN (Hardcover): 978-1-77204-530-7

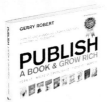

Publish a Book & Grow Rich
How to Use a Book as a Marketing Tool & Income Accelerator
Gerry Robert
ISBN: 978-1-77204-546-8

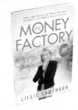

The Money Factory
How Any Woman Can Make An Extra $30,000 To $100,000 Passive Income
Lillie Cawthorn
ISBN: 978-1-77204-420-1

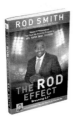

The Rod Effect
Master 8 Philosophies That Took Me from the Projects to NFL SUPER BOWL STARDOM
Rod Smith
ISBN: 978-1-77204-254-2

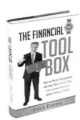

The Financial Toolbox
Your Best Business Guide To: Less Tax, Greater Profit And More Time!
Jessie Christo
ISBN: 978-1-92741-199-5

POWERED BY

www.blackcardbooks.com

OTHER BOOKS RECOMMENDED BY BLACK CARD BOOKS

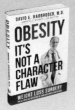

**Obesity:
It's Not A Character Flaw**
Weight Loss Surgery
The Alternative When You're
Done With Diets (And Blame)
David E. Hargroder, M.D.
ISBN: 978-1-77204-033-3

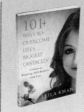

**101+ Ways to Overcome
Life's Biggest Obstacles**
A Guide to Handling
ANY Problem with Ease
Leila Khan
ISBN: 978-1-77204-436-2

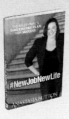

#NewJobNewLife
The Millennial's
Take-Charge Plan
For Success
Anastasia Button
ISBN: 978-1-77204-558-1

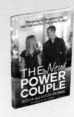

The New Power Couple
Designing an Abundant
Life and Relationship that
Lasts Forever
Jocelyn and Aaron Freeman
ISBN: 978-1-77204-635-9

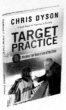

Target Practice
8 Mistakes That Ruin a
Love of the Game
Chris Dyson
ISBN: 978-1-77204-459-1

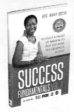

**Success Fundamentals
Vol. II**
Nuggets & Pearls of
Wisdom to Help You Pump
the Greatness in You!
Adv. Mary Bosiu
ISBN: 978-1-77204-437-9

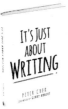

**It's Just about
Writing**
Peter Cher
ISBN: 978-1-77204-262-7

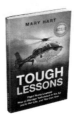

Tough Lessons
Flight Nurse Learned
How to Manage Turbulence
in the Air and in Her Life,
and You Can Too!
Mary Hart
ISBN: 978-1-77204-053-1

POWERED BY

www.blackcardbooks.com